Praise for

An Arrow Through the Heart

Designated a most outstanding consumer health title of 2002 by *Library Journal*

"Reads like a gripping suspense novel . . . A moving story in the face of sudden catastrophe; recommended for all health collections." —*Library Journal*, starred review

"*An Arrow Through the Heart* is an epiphany for women who mistakenly believe they are immune from the ravages of heart disease. Using her heart as a magnifying glass, Deborah Heffernan provides readers with a window into their souls." —Mehmet Oz, M.D., television talkshow host, cardiac surgeon, and Vice-Chair and Professor of Surgery at Columbia University

"For anyone who still lives with the illusion that heart disease belongs only to men, *An Arrow Through the Heart* is a shocking wake-up call. Heffernan takes you to the precipice and lets you stare over the edge of losing it all. From the mundane sweetness of ordinary days to the gut-wrenching emergencies, you go on the roller coaster with a woman who isn't supposed to be living this life. But she is . . . and what you learn along the way will change you." —Nancy L. Snyderman, M.D., chief medical editor, NBC News

"A commanding chronicle . . . Unmarred by self-pity, an arresting story that women and men suffering from heart disease will find, well, heartening." —*Kirkus Reviews*

"*An Arrow Through the Heart* is not only a book of hope and inspiration, it is also a journey of spiritual intrigue. The coincidences and synchronicities that the author shares within the pages of her life story hint in such a comforting way that heaven walks with us each step of the way in each moment of our lives. This book is magnificent."
—Caroline Myss, author of *Sacred Contracts* and *Anatomy of the Spirit*

"Nail-biting, almost cinematic suspense . . . This is an absorbing book. Well written and informative . . . it has much to offer as a reminder of the value of preparedness and of appreciating each day." —*Booklist*

"When one human triumphs against great odds, we are all lifted up. So we are with Deborah Daw Heffernan's encounter with heart disease. This is a heroine's journey—the story of one who braved everything, acquired wisdom and meaning, and returned to share with the rest of us." —Larry Dossey, M.D., author of *Healing Beyond the Body* and *Reinventing Medicine*

"Insightful and openly emotional." —*Publishers Weekly*

"Reading about catastrophe is always a dilemma: how can you enjoy a book about someone's physical suffering? But here you follow the example of Heffernan, who enjoys herself in odd, articulate, and hard-won ways. The Dalai Lama is rumored to giggle a lot, and you get the idea that this author wouldn't hold anyone's guffaw against them. Sublime humor, that high defense, is on the list of treatments she has picked." —Elissa Ely, M.D., lecturer on psychiatry, Harvard Medical School Bulletin

"I couldn't put it down! The truth shown like a torch on every page. There is nothing false, exaggerated or preachy here . . . [Deborah Daw Heffernan] does not make out her doctors to be Gods who treat her like a mere female child, but [as] experienced experts in a field she didn't know much about but wants to, who answered her constant questions without condescension and respected and trusted her knowledge of her body. She also describes her doctors as people with very human traits. I would recommend this book to anyone—colleague, friend, or patient. [An] essential book for women . . . to think deeply about and to re-evaluate your own life for a long time." —Dixie Mills, M.D., Association of Women Surgeons

"[*Arrow*] is as cathartic to read as it must have been to write. Heffernan makes no bones about the fact that part of the reason she wrote the book was to bring awareness to women of the little-known statistic that women are more likely to die of heart failure than anything else. So the book is in part a plea to women to take care of their health, both of the mind and the body, and to understand the warning signs and symptoms of heart attack . . . On the flip side the book is as personal a story of a year of someone's life as you could possibly read. Here is a woman who, in a moment, left the world of airports, cell phones, and meetings for a world where it took all her focus and strength to brush her teeth on her own. She forsook the world before her heart attack for the peaceful, slow-pace life in western Maine she had truly wanted all along. Forced to become mindful of every breath (literally and figuratively), to become almost completely reliant on her husband, family and friends, and to appreciate each day as the day her life could end, Heffernan eloquently describes her transformation to a peaceful, spiritual, and thankful existence." —Lucysbooks.com

AN ARROW THROUGH THE HEART

An Arrow
Through
the Heart

One Woman's Story of Life, Love, and
Surviving a Near-Fatal Heart Attack

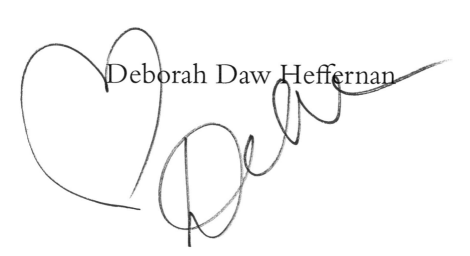

Deborah Daw Heffernan

The author gratefully acknowledges permission from the following sources to reprint material in their control: Arcade Publishing for text from *Dreams of My Russian Summers* by Andrei Makine, copyright © 1995 by Mercure de France, translation copyright © 1997 by Geoffrey Strachan.

Cover design and illustration by Honi Werner

ISBN: 978-1-5040-0921-8

Distributed by Open Road Distribution
345 Hudson Street
New York, NY 10014
www.openroadmedia.com

For Jack

and in loving memory of
Robert Kindellen Daw
December 21, 1912 – November 17, 2000

Contents

An Arrow Through the Heart

Illness is the night-side of life, a more onerous citizenship. Everyone who is born holds dual citizenship, in the kingdom of the well and in the kingdom of the sick. Although we all prefer to use only the good passport, sooner or later each of us is obliged, at least for a spell, to identify ourselves as citizens of that other place.

—Susan Sontag, *Illness as Metaphor*

By now she knew that this life, despite all its pain, could be lived, that one must travel through it slowly; passing from the sunset to the penetrating odor of the stalks; from the infinite calm of the plain to the singing of a bird lost in the sky; yes, going from the sky to that deep reflection of it that she felt within her own breast, as an alert and living presence.   —Andrei Makine, *Dreams of My Russian Summers*

Prologue

STATISTICS ARE AERIAL PHOTOGRAPHS. The photographer in the airplane circling high above us looks for the big picture—where land gives way to water, where mountains rise, where the desert begins. There is nothing to distract him from the landscape, no movement telling of life below the treetops. Yet we are there nonetheless, waving, waving, each with our own story, each with a heart whose beat gives us life and makes love a possibility.

When *An Arrow Through the Heart* was first published in 2002, the aerial photograph showed that cardiovascular disease (also called heart disease) was the number-one killer of men *and women* in the United States. The *women* part became BIG NEWS, and this little book joined an awakening medical and activist community in raising awareness that each year 2.5 million women were hospitalized and about 500,000 died from heart disease—more female fatalities than from all cancers combined.

Today, heart disease kills about 430,000 women, yet it continues to reign as women's number-one killer, still slaying more women than all cancers combined. If that doesn't get your attention, consider this: ten times more women die of cardiovascular disease than of breast cancer, which claims 40,000 women annually. Clearly cardiovascular disease is not solely a man's problem. And we women have to look deeper than our breasts and into our hearts.

The slight decrease in women's cardiovascular deaths today is largely due to faster detection and treatment—thanks to persistent education and awareness campaigns led by the National Institutes of Health (*Heart Truth/Red Dress*, launched in 2002) and the American Heart Association (*Go Red for Women*, launched in 2004), as well as pioneering advocacy from independent groups like WomenHeart (The National Coalition for Women with Heart Disease, founded in 1999).

Then came the 2002 *Oprah Winfrey* show about the shocking prevalence of young women experiencing heart attacks. I was joined on that show by several other young, female cardiac victims who very personally drove home the news that cardiovascular disease is not just an old lady's issue, either. The lovely producer who traveled from Chicago to film Jack and me at our home in Maine, later reported that *Oprah* received three million emails immediately following that show, her largest response until then. Furthermore, at least two women's lives were saved within minutes of the broadcast, because they had recognized the symptoms and received swift help.

Even with *Oprah*'s magic, however, current data from the Centers for Disease Control and Prevention shows that cardiovascular disease remains the leading cause of natural death among *young* women, ages 25 to 44—well ahead of breast cancer and second only to accidents and adverse events like cyclones and murderous boyfriends. Unlike men, most women who die suddenly from a heart attack have never exhibited any previous symptoms until that moment. Yet many doctors still do not prepare women to recognize the signals of a heart attack—especially not young women who seem to be in good health. Like I was, when one of my coronary arteries spontaneously dissected (tore) in a gentle yoga class, triggering the heart attack that nearly ended my life.

Yet despite national and local awareness-building efforts, women of all ages persist in denying that heart disease means YOU and ME! The American Heart Association tells me that only one in six American women believes that heart disease is her stalker—even though 90 percent of women have one or more risk factors for developing it. What is especially perplexing about women's denial is that this is one disease over which we have considerable personal control. Simple, healthy meals and a daily walk are hardly difficult pills to swallow.

Now consider this. Even though *more women than men* die from cardiovascular disease, women comprise only 24 percent of participants in heart-related studies. Clearly we do not know enough about how a woman's heart works, as any corny love song can tell you.

So listen up. Today cardiovascular disease claims one out of every three of us—one woman every minute of every day—whereas breast cancer kills one out of every 30. Think about this for a minute. Imagine meeting two cherished friends for a cup of afternoon tea. Which one of you will it be?

I bet you want me to join that tea party. Because I was almost a statistic and maybe "almost" is enough to exempt you and your beloveds, right? I would do that for you if I could, but only you can memorize the signs of a heart attack and pay attention. Only you can honor your precious life by eating your vegetables and exercising even a little bit every day—habits that ultimately prepared me for the fight of my life.

When death came for me on May 12, 1997, I was a healthy forty-four-year-old with no family history of heart disease; in fact, one grand-aunt had lived to a hundred and six. My annual physical had just confirmed my usual low blood pressure and low cholesterol. I'd never touched a cigarette, let alone smoked one. I was slender, exercised regularly, and ate all my vegetables. I even made whole-grain bread each week. I was *certainly* not a candidate for a massive, near-fatal heart attack, emergency open-heart surgery, and ventricular tachycardia (a deadly malfunctioning of the heart's electrical system). Neither would I have believed that I could be unconscious for eight days of my life. And I certainly never dreamed that a heart transplant would be in my future. I was in my prime, assuming my American birthright in grabbing cash from the ATM machine, throwing toothpaste and tomato paste into the market basket, and driving to work. Besides, I am a woman; I thought that in the matter of my heart's health, my gender would protect me. Wrong. Furthermore, only 50 to 70 percent of cardiac fatalities are caused by known risk factors. Since I had none of these, I belonged to the other half, people who are ambushed by heart disease.

A year and a half after my heart attack and surgery, on a flight to Anchorage, I met a cardiac surgeon from the Southwest who was recovering from open-heart surgery himself. I told him that I was drafting this book, and he said, "Even as a doctor who's prepared and operated on hundreds of patients in all circumstances, I had no idea what I was facing. Write your book for all of us. We need to understand more about what the patient goes through, from the patient's point of view."

And so I did. But my book is as much for families, friends, and people who deliver hospital breakfast trays and home heating oil as it is for patients and medical professionals. Matters of the heart cannot be separated from the muscle, I've discovered, so every person has an impact on the cardiac patient, who now believes that every moment is her last.

During my critical first year after being discharged from Massachusetts General Hospital in Boston, I found only a couple of books that offered the companionship and guidance I craved. There are plenty of books about fighting heart disease with diet and exercise, meditation and medication, but I wanted to know: *Is anyone in the universe like me—young, fit, female, shocked? What did you feel like? What happened to your life, to the lives of others close to you? How did you change, or did you not?* In the end, I've written the book that I searched for about heart disease. But it is also a book about facing catastrophic change of any kind and doing the work required for true healing.

As happens with most people who find themselves suddenly in what writer Susan Sontag calls the "kingdom of the sick," I grappled with cosmic questions after I had sought medical explanations. *Why me? Why my heart and not my toe? What could I have done to prevent this? Who is at fault?* My year's stay in the monastery of illness—a peculiar place of both confinement and release—took me deep into my past and I discovered that, as intuitive healer Caroline Myss writes, "Your biography can become your biology." While my biography is certainly not yours, perhaps like me you gain more from being swept up by the story of a real person's life than by a river of statistics.

The first year following a heart attack is the most critical period of recovery, a time when in closing your eyes at night, you can't trust that you will be there in the morning. Doctors struggle to prepare patients for this uncertainty, but there is no experience like personal experience. I have stuck strictly to that year and tried to be unflinching in my descriptions of the devastation, terror, joy, setbacks, insights, and unbelievable humor that accompany dying and returning to life again.

So come with me through five seasons in western Maine, where I recovered my body and soul. The first spring lasted only a month, yet I dwell on it the longest because after being given back life I observed it as fixedly as a child observes a bug. As the seasons progress, my descriptions of them shorten, reflecting my gradual return to healthy-people time—a time when a lemon drop no longer demands full attention until completely dissolved. We cannot meet our worldly responsibilities, which I did not for more than a year, while paying rapt attention to every raindrop on the windshield.

Simply by slowing us down, disease can tell us what our souls need to know. It becomes a diagnostic tool for the spirit. Difficult as that year was, I miss the languorous pace enforced by confinement. Driving thirty miles an hour no longer feels like speeding to me; I make lists of things to do and feel a tug if the day doesn't give me time to complete them; I occasionally walk by a flower without peering into it. But I doubt I will ever be truly inattentive again. I emerged from that monastery seeing my broken heart in a whole new light—as a metaphor. It's ironic that a devastating attack on my literal heart brought healing to my spirit-heart. I now understand that healing and curing are two very different things.

My doctors told me that by the time I reached the one-year anniversary of my heart attack I would feel strong and confident again. And they were right. But I didn't believe them for even one minute, not when the act of eating a chunk of fruit took centuries as the sun rose in a chilly hospital room.

Ultimately, this book is not about heart disease at all, but about digesting that fruit.

SPRING

1

THERE IS A WEIGHT ON MY CHEST. Right between my breasts, pressing on my breastbone—as though the atmosphere ripped open a shaft from the heavens to me and the sky poured down onto this one spot. Observant, detached, slowing down, breathing carefully, I think with my body.

"I am having a heart attack," I say to Zoe, my yoga teacher.

I am in Cambridge, Massachusetts, lying on my back on Zoe's clean, polished floor looking at white walls and gleaming wooden window frames. The pressure on my chest has become very specific. It is bearing down now and revolving like a vise, cranking my chest tighter and tighter. I feel no pain, just curiosity. It is the alert, still curiosity of an animal at the sound of a footfall in the woods, of a child beckoned by a frightening stranger, of a bird that senses a change in the atmosphere before a storm hits. The pressure, the twisting continues. It is not going away. I am beginning to sweat.

Zoe is bending over me because she's been helping me improve a gentle yoga pose, Reclining Marīcyāsana. The idea, she says, is that with the shoulders relaxed and arms outstretched receptively, the heart is released and can ascend to radiance. It is one of yoga's warming poses.

But I am cold. I look at my hands. They are marble white. I sluggishly realize that Zoe has helped me sit up; I suddenly feel her small, strong hand supporting my back. Now I have the sensation of cold rivulets coursing down my arms, millions of discrete trickles running from my shoulders, over my elbows, to my wrists. Nausea rises.

"I am having a heart attack," I say again, this time with the calm, clinical finality that comes from absolute knowledge deep within my body.

For only a moment, my mind protests. *Give it a minute. It must be a muscle pull.* But Zoe does not second-guess me. Instead, she trusts the voice of my body and asks me what I want her to do.

"I want you to call 911. Tell them I need a cardiac team. Tell them to take me to Mount Auburn Hospital. My doctor is Barbara Spivak. I need a cardiologist waiting for me. Something is terribly wrong."

The icy rivers flow to my marble hands. *Take charge, take charge, take charge.*

The 911 guys lumber in with armfuls of equipment—thundering male steps echoing into a serene white room with three women in tights sprawled on a polished floor. Quickly assessing what is needed, they joke that when they got the call they thought "yoga class" was code for a cult. I laugh. Everything is fine if I can laugh. They would be stern if something were wrong. I am aware of how big they are, how slender my classmates. I am amused by the space men take up and reminded of my husband in the bathroom, obliviously standing in front of the mirror I was using while happily telling me a funny story about his trip to the dump. I like these guys.

They hook me up to machines. They put a tiny pill under my tongue. They ask me how I feel. Not great yet, but better because they are here, though it's harder to look inside my body when they distract me with light bantering. I am feeling happy in this moment. It must be a muscle pull.

I laugh with them and ask, "So, what do you guys think?"

"We think you're a very lucky lady."

Whew. Take two aspirin . . .

But the biggest one is all business now. He finishes his response gently, firmly.

"You're coming with us to the hospital."

They strap me into a chair and will not let me move by myself. I think they are cute and want to show off how strong they are. I feel cold terror suffuse my body, taking over as the tingling trickles flowing down my arms retreat. Or am I too scared to feel them?

Two men carry me out the door backwards. It is the summer view I had as a girl riding the tailgate of Dad's woody station wagon, the same view I had as a young woman teaching in the Swiss Alps, nauseated from sitting backwards on a train and vowing never to do that again. As they load me into the van, I wave to a child and an old man, reassuring them that everything will be all right. Zoe's face is small and serious on the steps. I thank her and wonder at my self-possession. But I am simply *here*, in the arms of these funny strong men. Surrendering my independence, I feel a rush of relaxation.

Or am I deciding that I am relaxed when what is actually happening is that my body is failing me? What does that feel like? How would I know?

The men in the front seat are calling in to the hospital. I strain to hear what is said, muffled code words through glass. The big guy is still with me, administering more tests, asking me over and over how I feel. I no longer know. I desperately want to tell him that every test makes me feel better, but it does not, no matter how hard I try to please him. He shows no elation or disappointment. I can't read him. How am I?

I was dying of a massive heart attack, or myocardial infarction (MI). Between my first sensation of pressure and the rescue team's arrival, only ten minutes went by. Those ten minutes—an eternity—saved my life. I relive every second again and again. I think of all the places I could have been instead of within the serene walls of a yoga studio.

I was your typical harried working-woman, a partner in a small but prominent corporate training company. May 12 had been a Monday like any other—better than most because there was no packed suitcase behind my office door ready to be loaded into the four o'clock cab to Logan Airport, flung into another rental car in the evening darkness, and unzipped in another hotel in another strange city of blinking lights, with highways lacing it like a sneaker. As it happened, a client had called on Friday and switched our meeting to a phone conference later in the week. So on this Monday, instead of flying to Detroit, I was going to my yoga class and sleeping in my own bed next to my husband, the love of my life.

What if, bored and imprisoned in an airline seat a few months before, I hadn't picked up the in-flight copy of *Fortune* and read an article on heart attacks that described many of the symptoms I would experience? What if my Detroit client had not changed our meeting to a phone conference? What if I'd taken that one last call and been sitting in rush-hour traffic instead of in my yoga class focusing on my breathing, deeply attuned to my body?

What if I had reacted to my body's signals with denial and hubris? What if I had not acknowledged death in the moment it visited me?

I would be dead. And if I had died, I would not be *here*. I would not be looking up the lake at another spring, one year later, from my study in our old house in Maine. I would not be seeing our beloved Mount Washington across the border in New Hampshire, with snow lingering in Tuckerman Ravine like icing on the cake saved for last. I would not be listening to water lapping at the peninsula—each year an exciting new sound after the silence of ice stretched shore to shore during Maine's long winter. I would not be hearing the wind chimes on the northwest corner of the house heralding several days of blue skies and sparkling water. I would not hear the loons or the mourning doves or the tree swallows busily nesting in the fantasy birdhouse, made by friends for our wedding, with a brass heart for a weathervane.

Every day I am aware of my good fortune and regard each moment of life as the exquisite miracle that it is. I am also aware that before IT happened, I had lived each day as best I could—often too intensely, but always fully participating in life. As I write that, I pause. True? I will always wonder what I could have done differently. Did I appreciate life enough? Could I have prevented IT from happening?

With time, I am learning that the physical *why* is not important. That ride across Cambridge in the rescue vehicle with my burly boyfriends was the beginning of my journey of the heart in both the physical and spiritual sense, because I believe that to heal the body you must heal the spirit. With time, I have been able to see my catastrophic heart attack as the gift that it was.

2

IN THE EMERGENCY ROOM I am a magic trick, a rabbit who suddenly appears from under a hat as they lift me out of my chair and onto a bed in a room filled with beds. I do not remember entering the hospital with the 911 guys.

"I can do this," I tell them cheerfully, and assert life itself by rolling onto the bed unassisted, sort of. I hope they can see that I am fine if I can move like that. I was in my yoga class, after all.

Someone removes my sneakers. How did they get on my feet? I was barefoot in class. An elderly lady wearing a faded hospital johnny stares at me from the bed opposite mine. She looks scared, poor thing. It doesn't occur to me that she is staring in horror at the state I'm in. So I give her an encouraging smile as they crisply pull the curtains around me, the metal rings screeching along the ceiling rod like a car braking before a crash. My big boyfriends disappear and I feel like a lost child. No one is teasing me here. They hook me up to a heart monitor and I realize that something is seriously wrong, that I am in real danger.

Snow is beginning to cover me—softly, gently. I love the snow; it does not frighten me. I am deeply centered and practical.

"Please call my husband. Now. Jack Heffernan. Genzyme meeting at the Algonquin Club. Tall, silver-haired, handsome." I see his smile floating in the air like the Cheshire Cat's.

The busy people in green do not acknowledge me. They are all over my body, and I can tell my voice is not their priority—a new and disconcerting experience for someone who has worked for fourteen years as a consultant and whose advice is sought. I repeat my request, unsure whether I am actually speaking out loud. A doctor with a full beard looks up from the machine.

"You are our first priority, Mrs. Heffernan."

But I am steely; he has met his match. And I am remarkably lucid, still managing the situation as if I had spent my whole life preparing for it.

"Thank you. I know you are doing your job, Doctor, but not everyone in this room is attending to me. Someone must call my husband now." Thinking that as medical people they would be concerned about danger to him, too, I add, "Jack is a mountain climber and has been through a lot in his life. He's in biotechnology and understands medicine. He'll stay calm. Please call him."

Jack is bending over me. Such a lovely sight, such a handsome man. His brown eyes look concerned, but I choose to look at his smile, smooth pink lips stretched broadly over his strong white teeth. He is all dressed up in one of his corporate outfits, but I know that he pees in the pine needles the minute we arrive in western Maine every Friday night, where an old gray house sits waiting for us on a small lake. Jack is my love and he is bending over me. I smile back. But just as I open my heart to him, a knife slams into it—then nothing.

I have been to Nothing. It is a place. I remember it.

Jack jerks back the curtain and motions to the doctor as I fall back, my hands reaching for my chest. The doctor checks my heart readings and swiftly pulls the curtain around me again.

"Mr. Heffernan, we have to ask you to step outside."

People in green slip into my tent like raiding Bedouins. Jack, his eyes pleading, touches my hand to steady himself and then retreats behind the pastel curtain, now as impenetrable as a prison wall. We've always believed that we are the lovers Plato imagined: originally one person, the two parts having been separated and desiring to be joined again, no matter what. After all it took to find each other, we are being torn apart once more, and Jack is alone just when he needs me the most—seeing over and over again my hands flying to my chest, my face turning white, my gaze looking inward and away from him as I head for another world.

It took only a second for me to go.

We first met in a conference room much like the one Jack just left. He had invited my training company to Stamford, Connecticut, to present our services at GTE Corporation (now Verizon) headquarters, where he was the vice president of corporate human resources. After almost ten hard years helping to build our company

18

from one typewriter to twenty-five people, I was thrilled to be at GTE and trying my best not to show it. But crawling under the table to plug in an overhead projector, I hit my head with a loud thump and tore my dark stockings. I tried to hide the ribbon of white running crazily down my leg by walking sideways like a crab from the screen to my notes. My foolishness was confirmed by the wide grin on Jack's face. In spite of my rattled presentation, GTE sent us to work at various sites around the country. A year later I offered to take Jack to lunch as a thank-you gesture. Somehow the lunch was changed to dinner. I brought a briefcase containing my next sales pitch. Five hours later the briefcase remained untouched, and we hadn't even noticed the waiters piling chairs on the tables around us. Usually ravenous, I hadn't eaten a bite.

As in all adult courtships, we brought with us our histories. Jack's included a divorce and five children ranging in age from mid-teens to late twenties. Wisely, he "forgot" to mention the kids until our fourth date, by which time he could tell I really liked him. He told me carefully over dinner in my rent-controlled Cambridge apartment, and like any self-respecting woman, I promptly threw him out for misrepresenting the situation. At the bottom of the stained linoleum stairs with metal treads, in the flamingo-pink foyer with a gaping hole punched through the plaster, he tripped over my "car"—a beat-up, brown, three-speed Raleigh bicycle. Jack vowed never to talk to me again.

My history, on the other hand, included feeding one too many meals to men who were passing through before marrying someone else. It came to a head in the mid-1980s, when a speeding black BMW with a so-called "eligible young bachelor" at the wheel nearly flattened me and my Raleigh. I took it as a sign that maybe marriage was not going to be my fate; the man I wanted, who had both a career and a conscience, did not exist. I decided that I was content on my own and happy to listen to National Public Radio while putting up sauce with tomatoes from the Haymarket. Besides, friends were always eager to eat at my table; though I was single, I never felt alone. It was a good life. A divorced man with five kids was not what I needed. I was sick of taking care of other people's kids. I wanted my own.

But Jack's goodness haunted me. Watching him march down my linoleum stairs, rigid and wounded, I knew he'd be back and would never leave.

After a whirlwind courtship that felt short to everyone but us, we became engaged during a December whiteout on Mount Washington and were married one year after that restaurant meal I never touched. He was fifty and I was about to turn thirty-seven. When I told my father that I loved Jack Heffernan, five children and all, he looked at me as though I'd just told him I had breast cancer, and then begged me to quietly elope rather than embarrass him with a wedding. But his habit of supporting me prevailed. There is a photograph of Dad grinning happily at our reception, jacket off and tie askew after dancing all night with as many women as possible. But even as he came to love Jack, and believe in Jack's love for me, Dad would always be wary and ready to rescue me in the big old woody station wagon he still owned, in case any of us needed to move again. And my four sisters and brother followed suit, never getting too close, never really trusting that a man could love a Daw girl like our father always would.

Jack's children chose not to attend the wedding. I couldn't blame them. Being young adults did not make it any easier for them to sort out their feelings following their parents' divorce. Knowing many couples in second marriages, I have concluded that there is never a good time for a divorce and remarriage. No matter how civil or mutually consensual the divorce is, no matter how many years the marriage has been over, nor how relieved both parents and even children may feel, divorce rocks kids of any age because we always yearn for the perfect happiness we think other families enjoy.

Jack quit his job in Connecticut and moved into my three-room apartment. He didn't bring much with him. I cleared out a file drawer for his socks, shirts, and underwear. His few suits fit nicely in my armoire and we piled our sweaters together in my tiny closet.

With amusement, Jack discovered my peculiar relationship to technology. I could never find a flashlight with working batteries when I needed it, *plus* I had heard that batteries would keep well at low temperatures. Solution: Keep a loaded flashlight in the freezer! He found it when reaching for an ice cube tray.

20

It gets worse. Long before I met Jack, my friend Steven invited me to watch a movie on this new machine called a VCR. Thrilled, I went shopping for one the next day. The salesperson patiently spent an hour helping me find the perfect model. Triumphant and exhausted, he was about to excuse himself when I innocently inquired where the screen on the VCR was. I didn't own a television; I thought I wouldn't need one. After he stormed off in disgust, I left the VCR by the cash register and fled, mortified. Shortly after we married, Jack bought a TV in readiness for the Olympics and I didn't register its presence for weeks.

I discovered that Jack swirls his peppery-smelling shaving cream into an inviolable cone shape each morning, that he cries even more easily than I do, that he cannot get through the day without devouring the *New York Times,* and that he makes long, sentimental toasts at dinner while the soup grows cold and guests sneak sips of wine. I also discovered his enveloping calm, even when he was just beginning a job search in Boston and we had no idea how we would pay for college tuition and alimony.

Jack was never calm about missing his children, though. They were locked in a dance of approach and retreat that is common to all families affected by divorce. No one's fault, really. Just human beings stumbling around, trying to do the right thing, everyone hurting. Inside, I struggled terribly, though, trying to be patient and objective with Jack's kids so I could give him the best support—while also trying to understand my complicated family, with our own slings and arrows.

And then, one evening in our eighth year of marriage, I went to my yoga class, lay on the floor for my weekly release from stress, and felt my heart explode.

"We're taking her to the cath lab immediately for angioplasty," the bearded doctor emerges from my tent to report. "There are chairs in the hall outside the lab, Jack. We'll meet you there."

Sensing my gurney in motion, I am *here* again—just for a minute. I see the furry, intent face of the doctor. He is very close to me. I feel for him because I am helplessly sick and it's all up to him now. He has my complete trust.

I say, "I know something is very wrong. You must understand that if my bell is rung tonight—" *Why am I using that expression? I never use expressions like that. Always the editor, even as I am dying. I know I am dying. "*—it's okay. I have led a more beautiful and adventurous life in my forty-four years than most people have in eighty. I am very happy. You just do what you have to do."

The beard twitches and tilts down toward me. I realize that he thought I was asleep, so I grin, pleased that my voice is working and that I have set him straight.

"Mrs. Heffernan, as far as I am concerned, you are going nowhere."

In reality, the bearded doctor is long gone and a clean-shaven male nurse is attending me. Jack sees me mouthing words as though I have a thick wad of cotton on my tongue. I am talking to someone, but nothing comes out.

As instructed, Jack waits outside the catheterization lab on a vinyl-cushioned chair with chrome arms. A slight tear in the vinyl digs into his leg, but he doesn't feel it after the first prick. He sits up straight, watching the clock, waiting, both our lives in the balance. Nine o'clock, nine-thirty, eleven, twelve, two. In the end he is totally alone; even the cleaning people have gone home.

We are separated by a polished beige linoleum corridor, but Jack will later tell me that he did not see the floor at all. Instead he sees the cold and uncrossable glacial river that had rebuffed him, alone and dying, on a mountain in Argentina. Once again, he reaches for the calm and resolve he practiced twelve thousand feet above sea level to keep himself alive. Both our lives depend on it now.

Meanwhile, in the cath lab there are problems. The doctor is attempting to perform an angioplasty to open a major blockage in my LAD (lateral anterior descending artery). Speed counts: quickly opening a blocked artery prevents heart tissue from dying and may eliminate the need for open-heart surgery. But the angioplasty is not working and I am becoming even more unstable.

Awake and fascinated by the fluoroscopy screen for one brief moment, I watch the progress of the catheter, with its tiny balloon at the tip, as it passes through my artery. I do not realize how it got there, that an incision has been made in the top of my leg into which the tube was slipped to begin its journey against the flow of blood and up toward my heart. It is my last image from my life Before.

3

AT 3 A.M. I was moved to the cardiac care unit. I was stable and unconscious. On doctor's orders, Jack drove back to our apartment to try to get some rest. He poured himself a big scotch and put it on the night table. It stayed there for days, golden, untouched—like the black pumps kicked off by the closet, the gym bag open on the bed, the note telling him I'd be back from yoga class at eight-thirty.

Jack stared at my pearl necklace hastily dropped on the bureau and saw instead his mother's rosary beads. He had assumed that I would outlive him, that instead of dying alone on a scree slope, he would die in my arms. What if I died now? What would he do? Who would he be? What music would he play at my service and what would he say? Jack tried to imagine living alone in our house in Maine, the center of our universe, and felt sick.

For him it all began at his dinner meeting when a waiter appeared discreetly at his elbow and said Jack had a phone call. Jack pushed his chair back quietly, puzzled and suspicious.

How does he know who I am?

When a doctor with a foreign accent told him that I had had a heart attack and to come to Mount Auburn Hospital in Cambridge, Jack felt only disbelief.

"Surely this must be a mix-up. Say my wife's name again."

"Deborah Daw Heffernan."

"Again?"

"Deborah Daw Heffernan."

Jack put down the receiver in a dream. He composed himself quickly with an old trick that worked for jitters before giving speeches: he squeezed his toes together, imagining that they were in Maine soil. As an officer of Genzyme Corporation in charge of human resources,

Jack made a lot of speeches. But as he approached the conference room door, seemingly unruffled, inside he had begun to scream. He walked within a bubble that muffled the sounds of business-as-usual. Scanning the faces of his fellow officers and his own empty seat, he lowered his head and whispered politely to his friend the chairman, Henri Termeer.

"May I see you outside for a moment?"

In the corridor Henri protested, "Are you very sure Jack? It must be something else. How bad is it?"

"They didn't say. I-I have to go," Jack stammered, as if he were asking permission, always courteous, always deferential, clinging to normalcy.

"I'm coming with you!"

"No, Henri. Thanks, but no. I'll need you later," Jack said, knowing instinctively that something terrible was beginning.

Henri went back into the room and whispered to Dr. Rich Moscicki, Genzyme's chief medical officer and an immunologist at Mass General Hospital. As Jack raced down the stairs, Rich was right behind him. Our beat-up Subaru station wagon was sitting right out front, ready for the getaway.

"I'm coming with you."

"No," Jack said, "I can do this." Just as I had climbed onto the hospital bed unassisted, Jack's solo scramble into the car asserted that everything was fine, that he could manage this and it would all disappear. To allow Rich to come along would have been a dangerous acknowledgment that he was losing control.

He began to pull out onto Commonwealth Avenue, then slammed on the brake and leaned across the seat to the window. Rich came running to the side of the car.

"Rich, how do I get there?"

Having slept fitfully for only three hours on Wednesday morning, Jack got out of bed at 6 A.M., the untouched glass of scotch glistening on the night table. His experience as an expedition leader kicked in, and he coolly wrote down his communication plan. In spite of his emotional chaos, Jack was clear that he could not go through this alone.

He needed to hear himself say what was happening out loud for it to become real, for him to wake into the nightmare. So he called his eldest daughter in Great Barrington, Massachusetts, first, the child most like him in adventurous spirit and can-do attitude. Mary Kate had been up for an hour, the mother of four young children. Trained as a pilot and a nurse (because you never know when you might want to move to Alaska), she quickly got the facts.

"I'm coming right away, Dad."

He suddenly felt only panic. He needed his children desperately, but if they came, our two families would meet for the first time—over a hospital bed—in our almost eight years of marriage. My family had pretended that Jack's kids did not exist, and for a long time Jack's kids had pretended that I did not exist. He resented being torn like this now. No thank you, he would deal with the situation alone, keeping these planets with their own complex dynamics separate.

"Not until I know more, Kate."

"No, Dad. I'm coming," she said with finality. "I'll be at Brenda's. We'll call you at the hospital from there."

Mary Kate took charge of her father and then she took charge of the Heffernan family, calling Brenda, her youngest sister who lived in Boston, and then Meghan, Maura, John, and their mother, Brenda, a devout Catholic who began to pray and never stopped.

Next, Jack left messages at both our offices and alerted our Maine network of friends through Bob and Sally, who set up a phone chain. He reached our friend Juliana at her Beacon Hill home before she left for the office, and she called the old gang with whom I'd stumbled into careers and feasted on pasta and cheap wine. He left a message for Steven at his New York office because it was the only number he had. Steven had grilled Jack more sharply than my own father when he learned that I was in love with a divorced man with five kids—a gray-suit who climbed mountains, a villain not to be trusted.

Later in the day Jack would call his best friend, Morrie, in Seattle, the climber who had saved his life on Mount Aconcagua in Argentina and whose strength Jack needed again. Morrie was on his way to Ireland on business. His wife, Michelle, began to track him as he made his way from Seattle to Dublin, finally locating him in Chicago in the United Airlines executive lounge, dressed in his usual attire: jeans, sneakers, a flannel shirt, and carrying his briefcase—a backpack containing a state-of-the-art virtual office. At the very moment that his name was paged, Morrie was holding his cell phone and listening to the ring of our home phone. Jack had simply been on his mind.

At 7:30 A.M. Jack called Dad, which he describes as the hardest phone call of his life. He knew that he was about to bring an eighty-four-year-old man back to a time of whispers and muffled weeping, a time from which Dad had spent his whole life trying to distract himself and his children. Still, Jack knew not to call one of my sisters. It was important that he speak man-to-man with the patriarch who had never fully trusted him because the love of an outsider—especially a divorced man with five children—could never measure up.

"How about those Yankees this weekend?" Dad was barely awake, but immediately lively. He never wastes time.

"How are you, Bob?"

"I'm great, Jackson, how about you?"

"I'm not so great, Bob, and I need your help. Are you sure you are fine?"

Dad's tone shifted. "Yes, Jack, what is it?"

"I'm going to need all the strength you can give me, Bob. Can you do that? I need you to be strong for me because I am not fine."

"Yes, Jack." Dad's voice was low and firm, breathing with Jack. He was ready for the worst, a divorce, ready to go on the attack, thinking, *My daughter is no second-hand rose, buster, not with me still around to protect her.* Instead, he heard the unimaginable.

"Deborah had a heart attack last night. We don't know how bad it is yet, but it's not good. I'm not doing very well with it, and I need your help." Jack's voice began to wobble dangerously. He needed Dad's support, and he also knew that being needed would energize a man whose strength was mainly in his spirit now.

Silence.

"Are you there, Bob?"

A pause. "Yes, Jack."

"Will you call your family for me, Bob?"

"What happened and where is she?"

Fifteen minutes later Dad called back. He'd been sitting at his desk, head in hands, trying to absorb the news.

"Tell me again, Jack. Tell me again what you just said."

4

MY MOTHER, "ANCY" SHEA DAW, was forty-four—my exact age as I lay dying in a Cambridge hospital—when she died of Wegener's disease. In the woods of central Massachusetts she left a devastated husband with a fledgling one-man real estate and insurance business and six children under the age of thirteen. Wegener's is a genetic pulmonary disorder so rare that fewer than five hundred people in the United States have it at any one time. Today drugs can keep it at bay, but in 1965 Wegener's was a mystery, often misdiagnosed as pneumonia.

Mother simply faded away. I remember when her smell changed, and how thin she was, blue veins beneath papery, translucent skin— sensory details of illness that are more eloquent for children than words could ever be. The disease was beginning to affect her brain when Dad stopped my visits. As the oldest child, I had been the only one allowed in the hospital to visit her toward the end.

Sometimes I see her now in the shape of my feet and ankles.

When Mother died on September 22, 1965, I was thirteen and Rebecca, the youngest, was three, with the other four strung between us like T-shirts on a clothesline, flapping in the wind. We each reacted in defining ways. In spite of my father's insistence that I would have a normal adolescence, I became filled with a glorious sense of responsibility, pulling top grades, joining clubs, and working after school while trying to keep all the details of our life the same. That meant baking Christmas cookies and gathering branches of white pines from the forest to decorate our mantel just as she had, militantly cleaning kitchen cabinets, enforcing nap times, sewing dresses for my sisters, and unraveling if nine-year-old Robbie forgot to take out the garbage.

The others bobbed in my wake, creating their own identities as best they could. We were simply surviving, though Dad distracted us masterfully with Christmas mornings so full of presents that you could not walk into the living room, with puppies that ran away and circuses that ended.

He raised us adamantly by himself. We grew up in a crowded three-bedroom ranch house surrounded by apple orchards, hills, and reservoirs. We ran free beneath the pine trees and always came home on time, though there were no curfews. A benevolent dictator and the first feminist I ever knew, Dad loved us fiercely—protecting, encouraging, reprimanding, and teasing us. He inspired us to become loyal, hardworking, accomplished adults. Our greatest fear was disappointing him, so we never did.

I always knew that I would not make it past forty-four. I also knew that this was pure hysteria. But I *knew*. I never told anyone except a therapist I saw for a couple of years in my early thirties. Why did I feel that I had to go with Mum in death instead of outlasting her?

"It's natural to feel that way," the therapist told me. "Children whose parents die can't imagine being older than the parent. They feel guilty to think that they might enjoy a longer life."

And this was true. When I turned forty-four on June 27, 1996, I had reached the witching hour, the age beyond which I could not imagine. Not even Jack knew of my terror. As I had been off and on for the previous year, I was sick with a severe bronchial cold, once again on the verge of pneumonia. My doctor had prescribed increasingly stronger antibiotics over the course of that year. She said that I was traveling too much on business, working too many hours too intensely, that I took too much on. But I looked at her: she had four children and was thin as a rail. So how was *I* to stop? What right did I have? Sure I was tired, bone tired, but I had made it to forty-four.

That November one of my sisters unearthed Mother's medical records. I was stunned by the similarities in our symptoms: could I have Wegener's? I went to a specialist at Massachusetts General Hospital, who spent two hours with me and then had me tested yet again for allergies. The diagnosis: an allergic reaction to dust mites. The nasal spray worked. My relief was infinite.

But forty-four was not over yet. I thought it was, but it wasn't. Jack stood in a window overlooking the Mount Auburn Hospital parking lot, beyond which rolled the Charles River, gray and swollen with spring rain. He did not know what he was looking at, or even where he was. He was simply turned in that direction and he stayed there, waiting. Over the next two days, beneath Jack's eagle's nest, our families arrived, mine first. He was not looking forward to this family reunion of total strangers.

About 10 A.M. Jack saw my father walking across the parking lot with his familiar side-to-side rocking motion, caused by the pain of an ancient ankle injury. He held a bouquet of daffodils in his fist as if it were the flag and he were leading a Fourth of July parade. Dad was fighting thoughts about another time, when *his* father-in-law had walked into the hospital and *he* was in the window, vacantly waiting. Dad told me later that he was trying to push that image away and replace it with one he liked better: a smiling me sitting up in bed, gushing about the sunny daffodils, my mother's favorites. My father did not want to see the unconscious body of his daughter, as far away from him as the love of his life had been when he last touched her.

Three of my sisters arrived around 11 A.M. Ann had come from New Hampshire and Leesa from Maine to join Callie in Ipswich so they could drive in together. Below Jack's perch they moved like sparrows; darting and converging. My youngest sister, Becky, arrived a couple of hours later from southern Connecticut, her small face pinched and pale. They each entered the waiting room tentatively, aware of our scarred history and rigid with fear. As he hugged each of them, Jack could feel the tension in their bodies.

As they were racing to the hospital, I had slipped into critical condition. The angioplasty on Monday night had not been successful and my lungs had begun to fill with blood and fluids. The medical team was working frantically to stabilize me. It was becoming clear that I would need to be put on a left ventricular assist device (LVAD), a mechanical pump that could do the work of my dying left ventricle. The LVAD is a two-and-a-half-pound titanium machine, about the size and shape of a portable CD player, which is implanted under the skin near the stomach to pump oxygen-rich blood out to the body, normally the job of the left ventricle. It was developed by a group of Massachusetts engineers and scientists in the 1980s to keep seriously sick and otherwise doomed heart patients alive while they waited for heart transplants. In 1997 two leading Boston hospitals had well-established LVAD programs, but the Mount Auburn doctors feared I would not survive the ambulance ride.

When my sisters walked into my room, they saw a thrashing torture victim staked to the bed where I was supposed to be. Her face and neck were swollen and bruised, her mouth pulled tightly to either side by supports in a grotesque child's taunting expression, and her tongue protruded beneath a tube coming out of her throat. Blood pooled in her mouth on either side of the tube, smearing her like war paint. Before the anesthesia had fully taken effect, a breathing tube was forced down my throat to keep me from drowning in my own fluids. Slowly they recognized me. Although my eyes were wide open, I did not seem aware of their presence, arms and legs flailing so violently that they'd had to tie me down. Becky's first thought was for my bad back. It was the only problem she could grasp. She looked for a pillow, then felt foolish.

My brother Rob arrived around 3 P.M. and walked toward the doors below Jack's lookout, stiff with tension. He went to Jack and stuck out his hand, his bottled-up emotions visible on his face. Jack pushed the hand aside and embraced him fully. Then Rob turned away quickly, an ostrich who believes that if you hide, no one can tell that you are hurting. We hadn't seen each other in several years. When he had learned that Mum was never coming home from the hospital, nine-year-old Robbie had raced into his bedroom. Dad sent me in pursuit and I found him crouched on his bed, pounding his head rhythmically against the wall. His skinny little body fought me as I tried to pull him away from self-destruction. Robbie hadn't gotten enough hugs in the years that followed, and mine was the last touch in the world that he wanted. Leesa followed him now into the hospital corridor and watched in silence as he paced back and forth across the corridor, bouncing between the walls, lost in thought, time-traveling.

When Rob had collected himself and returned to the room, Dad beckoned to him and crumbled into his son's embrace. Had there ever been a moment like this between Dad and Puppa—a moment when our strong, gentle grandfather let Dad console him? Waking suddenly one dark autumn night in 1965, I had seen the two of them in our backyard standing over an incinerator sending brilliant orange flames to the sky, burning Mother's clothes, or so I feared. Puppa then turned into the woods for a solitary walk, shoulders heaving. His messy man-sobs were rendered silent by the pane of glass between us. I had only just learned what it sounds like when a man cries. Dad had made unfamiliar gulping noises when he told me that Mum was dead, but I never heard him cry again. Thirty-two years later, in another hospital, this was the first time my younger siblings had ever seen Dad cry. It lasted only a moment.

5

"SHE MAY NOT MAKE IT, JACK."

Our beloved general practitioner, Dr. Barbara Spivak, held Jack in a close embrace and whispered in his ear. It was Tuesday afternoon and she had pulled him into a lounge, away from the family. Terror was ripping Jack apart like the wind that once shredded his tents on Denali. He began to sob on Barbara's shoulder and she cried with him. Each time they thought I had turned a corner, new complications arose. Jack alternated between seeming dazed and in command, so Barbara wanted to be sure he understood the severity of the situation.

"I want her to go to MGH, Barbara. Genzyme knows the doctors there..."

"And that is probably what will happen, Jack. But she is too unstable to transfer and I can't override the doctors here. When the moment comes, they'll know."

Jack didn't realize that since the minute his station wagon pulled away from a Commonwealth Avenue curb, his colleagues Rich and

Henri had worked all that night and into the next on a backup plan, conferring with the doctors at Mount Auburn Hospital and several other specialists, one of whom they tracked down on vacation. The discussions were fueled by desperation; there was no room for error. And, despite all his experience in health care, Henri was shaken to discover that world experts had vastly different opinions about what should be done.

They concluded that a dangerous transfer to Massachusetts General Hospital or Brigham and Women's was the only option. World leaders in cardiac care with LVAD machines, both hospitals were just across the Charles River, which separates Cambridge from Boston. Anticipating that MGH would be our choice because of its strong relationship with Genzyme, Rich had already begun to brief cardiologist Dr. Marc Semigran, and Marc in turn had begun briefing surgeon Dr. David Torchiana. In fact, I had already taken a place in the back of the doctors' minds as they made their rounds.

But Jack and our families knew none of this in the waiting room across the Charles River, a gentle, meandering boundary between despair and hope.

On Tuesday night Rob took my father home. My sisters decided to sleep on the floor of the waiting room. Pizza and sodas were delivered and the nurses brought blankets and pillows.

Barbara looked drawn. She approached Jack as everyone was settling down.

"You must go home now, Jack. It's doctor's orders. She is quiet now and in good hands."

He shook his head in refusal. Barbara persisted.

"I want everybody to hear this: Jack must get rest." Then she said softly, looking right into his eyes, "You will have many decisions to make tomorrow."

Jack shot her a look as if she'd slapped him. Her face was persuasive. He went home, seeking the privacy and quiet our doctor had prescribed.

On the kitchen counter he found the chicken pot pie I had taken out of the freezer to eat after my yoga class, floating in a puddle. He threw it away and cried. He prayed that the phone would not ring that night.

My sister Ann woke suddenly at 3 A.M. on Wednesday—alert, aware. She strode purposefully down the hall to my glass-walled room just as she used to march fearlessly through the crowds of the county fair for the mustard and ketchup we'd forgotten. She saw people in green swarming around me. The energy was charged.

One nurse happened to turn to her. "Thank heavens you came here. She's going. Call Jack."

Jack picked up the phone before the ring began. "Get here quickly, Jack," Ann sobbed. "They're losing her."

He flapped helplessly in circles for a few seconds, moving first in one direction, then another. *I've got to get a grip. I'll take a shower.*

People hold on to odd, civilizing rituals when crisis comes. Throughout our ordeal, Jack's rituals involved keeping himself meticulously groomed. *If I look good, everything is good,* he reasoned. This is a man who has one change of clothes in Maine, whose favorite navy-blue sweater is riddled with moth holes, and who once told me that there are two kinds of mountaineers, the ones who bring a toothbrush on month-long expeditions and those who don't. He doesn't.

Freshly showered and shaved in cold water and dressed for a board meeting, Jack left our apartment and pressed the elevator button frantically. Did the elevator always take an eternity to come from the first to the third floor? He considered the stairs, but knew he couldn't trust his legs. Instead, he began to scream.

"No, No, No, Nooooooooooo. Please Don't Take Her Away."

He shouted prayers to his father and my mother, begging them to exert influence with the gods. It was the middle of the night, but not a door in the building opened. He fishtailed out of the parking lot, then missed the "H" sign on Storrow Drive and had to figure out where he was and loop around. The emergency entrance was closed and he pounded on the door. A security guard let Jack in and led him swiftly through the hospital to find me hooked up to more wires than you'll see in the interior of a television set.

We have all had moments in life when we look back and say, "This was the moment when I could have chosen another path, but I did not." I could have believed that my twisting chest was a muscle pull and ignored it. Jack could have left everything up to the hospital. But he did not. He called Henri Termeer from his cell phone at 4 A.M. and Henri was ready for the call.

"Jack, it's already handled. Call Rich. He has the medical steps in motion."

Rich's wife answered the phone halfway through the ring. "He's been waiting for your call."

"We have two medical teams waiting for you, one at MGH and one at Brigham. You choose," said Rich.

"I can't choose. You're the doctor. *You choose!*"

"All right, MGH it is." Friendship broke the technical tie between these two fine hospitals. These were the doctors Rich knew best, men and women he'd trained and worked with. Rich's personal confidence in my doctors offered invaluable reassurance throughout our ordeal that everything was being done that could be done. We were very lucky in this because wondering about whether the chosen path is the right one or not can be torturous for families. Once we enter the doors of a hospital, most of us are completely out of our element. Trust is everything.

At the same time, the Mount Auburn team that had worked hard through the night had agreed that only an LVAD and eventual transplant would save me and had begun preparations to transfer me to Massachusetts General Hospital. Moving me in a dangerously unstable state was now worth the risk. When Barbara arrived early at the hospital, Jack told her that the transfer was under way. He felt strong and in charge again, knowing that he was delivering me into the best available hands. Then Jack went back to his sentry post at the window, alone in a place where no one else could come with him.

From the moment Jack and the hospital decided to move me to MGH, my sister Becky began to notice that with each horrid piece of news, another door of hope opened if she could only hang on for another ten minutes. She called it the "snooze button," inspired by her fondness for this option on her alarm clock. Throughout the ordeal

to come, she hit this button when her inner alarm went off. *Whack.*
Snooze. *Whack.* Snooze.

6

AROUND 8 A.M. ON WEDNESDAY, Jack's family began to arrive. Watching his daughters approach the same doors that my family had passed through the day before, Jack felt tension, then put it aside. He let go of responsibility for people's comfort and put trust in their dignity.

Mary Kate and Brenda, Jack's youngest daughter, arrived first, and then Meghan who may have spoken for her sisters and brother eight years before when she said through tears, "I'd really like you if you were not marrying my dad." Now Meghan was so radiantly pregnant with her first child that she could barely squeeze out of the car. Maura and her husband, Tim, who lived in Portland, Maine, made sure their teaching schedules were covered and began to pack up their two small children for the drive south. John kept in touch from New York City.

Mary Kate strode right into the room and hugged my father, shocking everyone. Disarmed, Dad suddenly blurted out his truth, held deep inside since the day I told him that I loved Jack Heffernan and he stared down at his mashed potatoes.

"I just want to say how sorry I am. That I don't believe in divorce. That I was not at fault."

My sisters looked stricken. Wings fluttered. Then Mary Kate mumbled something brilliantly soothing and the moment was absorbed. She seemed unfazed that Dad was absurdly seeking absolution for something wrought by her own parents. In these bizarre circumstances, it was no more incongruous than if someone had begun to sing.

I have come to realize that for Dad this was actually a reasonable thing to say. In the world he was handed by his wife's death, my father believed that a man's children come first. A man of deep yet iconoclastic Catholic faith, he even defended us against his beloved Catholic

Church. Our kindly parish priest once approached him at the Communion rail, where Dad was saying his penance for having done his best all week. Father Lynch tried to reason with him about my parents' decision to enroll me in kindergarten at the Congregational church, a program known to be creative and advanced. In the 1950s any good Catholic understood the risk of a small child straying into a Protestant church. She could burn in hell for wanting to see what it looked like. But Dad believed that God was more reasonable than this and he responded, "Father, I will build bridges in this town that you will one day walk across. The quality of my children's education comes first, always first."

So, though he'd made a point of never asking me anything about Jack's children, Dad had actually taken the Heffernan brood into his heart from the moment he learned that they were part of my marriage package. He worried for them because he deeply understood the impact of loss on the young. He also worried because he could not protect me from the anger he feared they would feel. Instead, he had to entrust my happiness to the father of those children, a man whose loyalties he feared would be divided. Dad had felt helpless, yet responsible.

I had misunderstood my father's silence. He had underestimated my husband. All this Dad had stored up until our two families met for the first time and he unburdened his heart to an unlikely confessor, a woman who had initially opposed our marriage as vehemently as he had.

Why is it that we will never fully know the grandeur of our parents, though we have observed them closely enough to see lines and creases form?

Meanwhile, my sisters and Jack's other daughters merged like the fingers of two hands in a warm clasp and were talking away in minutes. They liked each other. They *really* liked each other. A surreal party atmosphere took over, fueled by hope and hysteria over how long it was taking to prepare me for transfer to MGH. Our friend Juliana arrived just as the transfer was in high gear. She walked into pandemonium, with people pacing, talking at once, sobbing, Jack rigid and pale, his children in a ring around him. Ann, whom Juliana at first thought was a nurse, suddenly dissolved into tears about a stupid "fight" at Christmas. No, it had not been good between my family and me for a while. This heart attack was very badly timed.

"You should all get in your cars," a nurse announced. "She's coming out."

At 9:30 A.M. two families and Juliana formed a caravan of five cars, motors idling, lights on like a funeral procession. Jack and Brenda were in the lead car. She begged her father to let her drive, but he refused the loss of any more control. Relegated to the passenger seat, she put her hand on his knee instead.

Suddenly a buzzing human hive of green burst through the wide automatic doors of the hospital. Behind the steering wheel of his car, Jack's whole body tensed: he'd caught a glimpse of my body in the center of the hive, connected by a tangle of tubes and wires to several poles and machines that were being raced into the huge ambulance with me. They closed the doors, and gray glass separated us. Then the ambulance driver approached the driver's side of Jack's car.

"I just want you to know, sir, that it's illegal for you to follow me too closely. If I have to put on my siren, you may not follow me. You'll just have to get to the hospital on your own. I'm sorry, but it's the law."

May 14 was another cold, drizzly day, more like a morning in March. The sky churned with stubborn gray winter clouds as the caravan crossed the Charles onto Storrow Drive, which runs along the river's Boston banks. It was morning rush hour on one of Boston's main arteries—a time of blinking red brake lights, bleating horns, and scowling, white-knuckled drivers.

That day, not a car was on the road.

The ambulance never needed its siren. From the air the speeding cars might even have looked like a kite with a colorful tail swaying with the bends in the river, the first car closely following the ambulance in violation of the law.

At the Copley Square exit, Storrow Drive descends slightly into a tunnel. The ambulance tilted down and Jack's lights penetrated the smoked glass doors of the ambulance for a few seconds. He saw people in green busily hovering over me and a woman in a down jacket pumping my chest ceaselessly, as if it were a machine. She did not lift her head. He could see my face looking right at him like death.

As we pulled up to the emergency entrance of Mass General, another green swarm spun out of the doors, swift and elegant in their movements. Jack sprang from his car and a man stopped him.

"Mr. Heffernan, she's in good hands. There is nothing more you can do. Please go to the Ellison Building fourth-floor waiting room."

Jack stepped off the elevator for the surgical intensive care unit (SICU or Sick-U) into the open arms of our friend Sharon, who had set out from Maine at 6 A.M. Her embrace grounded him, embodying the extended network of people who had begun to ride this out with him from several corners of the earth.

7

AROUND 10 P.M. nine family members, Juliana, and Henri were summoned to a small room dominated by a large conference table to meet the medical team that had been working since morning to stabilize me and find a solution.

They were greeted by cardiologist Dr. Marc Semigran, a Harvard Medical School graduate and faculty member. A tall man built like a former linebacker, he loomed over Jack, who is six foot three. At the same time, he had the thick, curly hair and the dimpled rosy cheeks of a shepherd boy in a Renaissance painting. His tweed jacket was several sizes too small, making my sisters want to giggle.

Becky had met Marc by my bed only minutes earlier—talking to me in a slow, exaggerated voice in case I could hear him. He had called me "Debbie" and she came swiftly to my defense, knowing that names are anchors.

"Her name is Deborah," she said angrily. "*Deborah*. She won't know who you're talking to if you call her Debbie."

Marc made the correction courteously, always calm, always focused. Immediately Becky wanted to beg his forgiveness. But Marc wouldn't have known what she was talking about.

Now Marc began to draw my heart on a whiteboard with simple, sweeping strokes, as if he were drawing an engine. He is a sober man, a man who communicates facts directly, carefully, and honestly—a realist who deals in no conjecture. He explained everything as accurately as possible so that this intelligent group could participate fully. But there was no way around it: the shepherd was the bearer of very bad news, and even this group of determined optimists lost hope. "By the time he was done we had melted all over the floor," Juliana later said.

One of my main arteries, the LAD, had spontaneously torn, or "dissected," as Marc would say. Yes, there had been a clot, but had the dissection of the LAD unleashed the clot, or had the clot ripped the LAD apart? No one knew, but the end result was that my left ventricle was dying. And this was dire because the left ventricle—something most of us haven't given much thought to since tenth-grade biology— is the powerhouse of the heart. It pumps blood to the extremities and, most critically, to the brain.

Then the doors swung open and surgeon David Torchiana entered. When he saw the crowd waiting for him, he hesitated just a minute, as though he might flee at the sight of so many dazed, sad faces. (Most family meetings involve a couple of people and lots of space.) Then he moved to the front of the room with the grace and intensity of a pitcher and took charge of the atmosphere. "Torch" is also a graduate of Harvard Medical School and a faculty member. About Marc's height, with a large, rangy build, Torch has hands the size of a mechanic's without the calluses. His fine, straight brown hair flops over his forehead wherever the cowlicks twist it and his mustache droops, making him look perpetually sad, like Sonny Bono. My sisters pictured him with a long ponytail on a Harley, riding with impossible freedom across the country.

Though there really was no choice about what to do—and Torch had clearly made up his mind about what he *would* do—he worked his magic to be sure that the family became part of the life-saving team. There would be surgery and there would be prayers, and he wanted to be sure they held up their end of the bargain.

"We have two options," Torch stated flatly. "We can wait for her heart to stabilize and then do a transplant. But she might not survive the wait for a new, compatible heart—even though she would be at the top of the transplant list because of her youth and otherwise good health. The other option is to operate immediately, attempting a triple bypass. I recommend this option because of the risk involved in the transplant."

"What is the risk of the bypass, Doctor?" Jack asked, riveted. In that moment he was alone in the room with Torch.

"Fifty-fifty."

"What exactly does that mean?"

"She has a 50 percent chance of not making it out of the operating room, Jack."

Jack exited his body, perched in the corner of the room, and saw a dark future with no more Maine, no more travels, no more daily routines, no more teasing. . . . Then he felt someone rubbing his back and realized that he was still there, still gripping the table.

"And if it works, then what?"

"Most bypasses last ten years."

"Then what?"

"We go in again and redo it."

Jack considered this for a second. Then he pounded the table.

"I want twenty years!"

His daughter Brenda punched the air in a fierce, silent cheer. Electricity ricocheted around the room. Someone asked another question, and Torch moved into high gear, firmly yet politely.

"There isn't time for me to explain everything. Time is running out. We have to move right away. It's a long shot, but it's the only shot we have. I need a family decision quickly. Right now."

Torch looked penetratingly at Jack.

Not realizing at first that the decision was his alone to make, Jack looked at Dad. "With your permission, Bob . . ."

"Whatever you decide, Jack, I support it fully," Dad said, phlegm rattling in his throat. He had collapsed like a small Maine brown bat in daylight, shoulders slumped, head in his hands. Here, at last, he was thoroughly entrusting my husband with my well-being—a terrible and liberating moment for both of them.

Jack rose to his feet, but there was no earth beneath him. He levitated. Any suffering he had ever endured and any obstacles he had surmounted occupied the clouds beneath his feet. There were people sitting at a long conference table; there was a whiteboard. These absurd reminders of the corporate world put him in command again. He had his suit on. He was prepared, clear.

"I speak for myself, and I know I speak for my wife who has 'gone for it' throughout her entire life."

He saw me wearing an apron in the kitchen with pots simmering and three recipe books open. He saw me climbing Ben Nevis beside him in a whiteout. He saw me reading a book with fixed concentration, skating across the lake with the swift joy of an animal. He saw me zipping the suitcase shut and kissing him goodbye before the cab arrived at five in the morning, and beaming with delight when he surprised me at the airport upon my return. He saw this in a flash, and he knew what I would want him to do.

"Please operate immediately."

My sister Callie promptly fainted. Her building migraine had finally peaked. People in green surrounded her like luna moths drawn to a porch light just flicked on.

Jack never even noticed. He walked to the whiteboard. He held one of Torch's hands and touched his face, giving it three firm pats. "You do what you need to do, Doctor, and you bring my baby back. Bring her back to me."

"I'll do the best I can. But pray for us, Jack. We're going-to need all the help we can get."

Another doctor presented Jack with authorization papers to sign—pages of risks and consequences, all of them dire.

"I don't need to read this. I know," Jack said.

He had a flash of living with his decision if the procedure did not work, wondering too late whether he should have held out for the transplant. Then he carefully drew a heart with an arrow through it at the top of the page and wrote "I love you, baby. Come back to me." With confidence and relief that he had chosen the only route up the ice wall, that I was in the hands of the best, and that he had done all he could, Jack signed at the X. The doctor walked away with my life in a pile of papers. Then Marc and Torch disappeared like ground fog that is suddenly not where you were just looking.

Someone was rubbing Jack's back again, and he looked up and saw Henri nodding at him, eyes closed, deep in thought.

"It's the right thing to do, Jack, a bold and good decision."

Callie—my first sister and friend, my ingenious opposite who'd toppled my perfect sand castles and sabotaged my first date by giggling mercilessly behind bus seats—began to stir.

"There you go again, Cal, stealing Deborah's thunder," my sister Ann said.

Laughter seeped out like burps of nausea.

Within the hour I was prepped and ready to go. Dr. Greg Koski appeared, dressed in full scrubs, mask dangling beneath his beard, leading an army of green that was wheeling me to the OR on a gurney attached to bottles, tubes, and machines. The director of cardiac anesthesiology research, he had been called from his bed to join the team.

"Give her a kiss, everyone, give her a kiss."

They filed by shyly and kissed a woman they no longer recognized. She was Humpty Dumpty, a tube protruding from her throat, which was swollen to twice the size of her head, her body puffed with forty extra pounds in fluid, her tongue a black fish.

Jack followed the gurney with body and soul as I was pushed into the ambulance-size stainless steel elevator, the express train to the operating room.

"Give her another kiss, Jack," Greg said gently. Our families turned away, their teary blindness the only privacy they could offer in a stark and sparkling hallway.

Juliana rounded the corner at this moment, having just updated her husband from a pay phone. She saw Jack alone by the elevator as the doors slowly shut. *Whoosh, whump.* Silence. Under the harsh fluorescent lights, Jack hammered the air with his fists, yelling in a whisper.

"Fight, Deborah, fight. Fight it, baby."

8

MY FAMILY ONCE AGAIN CAMPED OUT on the waiting room floor. Dad was propped in a chair. Jack tried to sleep, then gave up. All night long he sat stiffly in a chair, elbows on knees, eyes on the clock, unaware that his youngest daughter, Brenda, had returned to the hospital and was holding vigil just outside the door. She'd tried to go back to her apartment in Boston's Italian North End but had been repulsed by normal life and a cold pizza on the kitchen table.

In the operating room, my heart and lungs had to be stopped completely for the bypass, and my cardiopulmonary functions were being maintained by machines. Marc left the operating room himself to tell Jack when the hookup had been successful. Almost every hour someone in scrubs, silhouetted by cold light from the hallway, would stand in the door of the waiting room and report. "She's still with us, Jack. It's still okay." So calm, so factual. At 2 A.M. a call came from the OR that they had successfully completed a double bypass. My heart was pumping blood and the internal bleeding had finally stopped. A balloon pump would be kept in my aorta for some time, however, to support my heart circulation.

Torch appeared at 3 A.M., decorated with a few drops of blood, his mask dangling from his neck. "She made it, Jack, and she's doing very well." He was pleased overall, but concerned about a deadly arrhythmia they'd fought during the operation. Six times the operating team had brought me back from death due to repeated episodes of ventricular tachycardia—a rapid, shallow heartbeat in the left ventricle that is essentially caused by a short in the heart's electrical system.

Torch explained that they had had to sedate me heavily to keep me quiet and flat, and that this would continue for several days because, sick as I was, I kept fighting the sedation that I needed to heal. As many days as I was under sedation, it would take at least that many for me to come back. He apologized for going home to get a couple of hours of sleep.

A nurse called from the SICU to say that Jack could see me now.

Becky and Leesa followed him while everyone else slept, utterly spent. They stared at my inert body, helpless. *Where are you, Deborah?*

At 7 A.M., just before making his rounds, Torch checked in with the family again, freshly shaved, a can of Coke and a clipboard in his huge hands. I was stable, I was holding on.

I am in a soft, warm cave, a chipmunk's den like the one in the stories my mother told me. I am small and happy. Occasionally I am *here*, moving up a long passageway to where the light is. Now someone is brushing my hair. I feel a hand on my forehead. Jack's voice. Then I hear Ann's voice, Leesa's voice. Why would they be here? I thought they didn't want to come to our house for Christmas.

Something is restricting my legs, something I want off, off, off. I am kicking furiously at massive weights tied to my feet and finally I am free. *Much better. Everybody out of my way.*

Someone is saying how nice my skin looks, that I belong in maternity, not in cardiology.

Cowgirl Cream.

I mouth my beauty secret as though there is nothing wrong. Somebody giggles. I hear them talking about shopping for sneakers for me. Ann realizes I am *here* again. She comes to the bed and voices my longing, "You want to come shopping with us, too, don't you, Deb?" I nod yes; I am sad to be left out. *I am always left out of their fun. It is not fun to be the oldest. And now they are all here just like I always wanted, but they're going shopping without me.* I am agitated and try to tell her how much I want to go, to be part of their bunch. She floats off and I am looking at Jack and me; we are smiling. I am peaceful, happy, I return to my cave and *nothing.*

These are the only memories I have from the eight days of unconsciousness that began when I passed out at Mount Auburn Hospital. Family and friends took turns by my bed for those eight days and four more while I came out of sedation—telling me the day and time, what had happened and that I was fine, identifying who they were, brushing my hair, smoothing my forehead, holding my hands. They told me funny stories, and that they loved me—keeping me alive when they could tell my spirit had burrowed deep. They talked to me as if I were all there. They explained that the weights on my feet were Air Jordans, laced to prevent drop-foot from prolonged inactivity in bed. (I kept kicking off the surgical booties strapped on by Velcro.) Ann and Leesa had purchased my Air Jordans on upscale Newbury Street, frantic to buy the best as a talisman. It was all they could do.

I remember none of this, but I felt it.

I keep searching my body for traces of those twelve days when only a photograph of Jack and me in Rome, held up to my nose, would quiet me. I remember no pain, so I have not even that to latch on to. As a child, I was fascinated by the story of Rip Van Winkle, a man who slept so long that when he woke up, the world had changed. I went to sleep, too, and my world changed abruptly, violently. This was not all bad; after all, my sisters were stroking my head and buying me shoes.

At 8 A.M., the morning after surgery, Dad is standing at a window, gazing into the sky. He is mad at God and letting him have it.

Not again. You can't take another one from me. I've worked hard. I've done a good job in raising all six of them, all by myself. You took my first love. You may not take my second.

Dad's potent contribution to modern medicine was to concentrate at that window, sending God messages of his disappointment—a sure crumbler for any of his children. He went in to look at me only once, preferring to send my sisters as emissaries to report back from the front. As the general, he remained focused on overall strategy, looking into the clouds above Boston.

In the meantime, the universe was arriving in the tiny SICU waiting room. Friends from near and far milled around. Baskets of food filled the place like a deli. The phone rang constantly, and Jack assured distant supporters that there was nothing they could do here, that we needed their prayers above all. Our Maine neighbor and electrician Joe had to unpack his van and pull his weeping wife, Arlene, from the front seat and back into their house to wait it out from afar. Jack's ex-wife called several times, causing my father's mouth to shape like a Cheerio as he considered the novel idea of people remaining friends after divorce.

45

Yes, people came out of concern for me, but mainly they came to support Jack, knowing that he would be seriously adrift. Our friend Steven recalls that "we all operated like one big muscle." The result was that Jack was surrounded by people distracting each other and taking care of practical matters like food and sleep so he could focus on me and fall apart occasionally. They took turns tapping into every emotional shift and were there to catch him. Nothing was hidden. Emotions were raw and often exploded into hysterical soliloquies. My sister Ann began to speak in one-liners like the tea mouse in Alice in Wonderland she once played charmingly in summer camp.

Dad hadn't seen many of our friends since our wedding and he became giddy with all the tragedy, fear, reunion, and laughter swirling in the room. He joined the fray, rambling on with jokes from his favorite sitcom until he collapsed. Rob wisely drove him home to rest.

Back in Maine, animists, atheists, and fundamentalists gathered on our property in a remarkable ecumenical effort to reach the gods. They filled a shoe box with tiny bags of fragrant soil and moss, a jar of lake water, a duck feather, spruce cones. Our friend Bob added a medicine spoon he'd carved in the form of a snake. His wife, Sally, wrote a beautiful poem. Someone took a Polaroid of the group holding a get-well sign in our driveway and put that in the box last, so it would be the first thing that I would see.

Frances Hodgson Burnett wrote, "When you have a garden, you have a future, and when you have a future, you are alive." My gardening friends conducted their own rites to ensure this. Lucia and her crew visited my garden to uncover tulips desperately pushing toward the sun from under their heavy cover of winter mulch. While I was trying to emerge from the drugs, Lucia's mother tucked in a few white campanulas that would bloom just about the time she estimated I'd come home, very much alive.

At Genzyme, Jack was overwhelmed by the outpouring of love both from people he worked closely with and others he barely knew. But they replied, "It's your turn, Jack. Let us take care of you for a change." And Jack surrendered with relief. He accepted the smallest favors, knowing that other people felt as powerless as he did.

46

Though unconscious, I felt all this love. It was a warm light wrapped around me in my cave, deep inside my body, miles beneath my skin.

9

JACK WAS LOOKING RAGGED and the doctors insisted that he go home to sleep. He wouldn't leave. So my sisters conspired: they would stay at the hospital twenty-four hours a day so he could return to our apartment and rest. They found a shower and learned when it wasn't used so they could sneak in. After several days of wearing the same clothes and not brushing their teeth, they went home to get a few things.

I have always found it interesting to see what people pack for a journey, especially small children. When Jack's grandchildren visit, their brightly colored backpacks contain magic sticks and stones, dead bugs, secret boxes, tiny dolls, favorite blankets, and floppy animals with most of their stuffing long gone. These items are simply indispensable on a trip to the unknown. Adults are no different when preparing for an uncertain journey. My sisters returned to the hospital with their own odd and very individual items, seeking comfort the way Jack had when he took a shower while I lay dying at Mount Auburn Hospital.

Ann pulled out a threadbare flannel nightgown with no elbows, a large yoke, and buttons down the back that's been her comfort uniform since high school.

"You're not really going to wear that," said Leesa, whose pronouncements rival Diana Vreeland's. In her business, decisions about featuring a pink or a blue shirt can make or lose thousands of dollars.

"Of course I am."

"Ann, don't be ridiculous."

"Well *you're* wearing sweats."

"That's the point, Ann. These are *sweats*. They disguise that I'm sleeping here. Your nightgown will blow our cover."

Ann deferred—it was easier—and slept in her clothes. But she leaned her head every night on that ratty old nightgown.

My husband stayed at our apartment for only a couple of nights. Neighbors, many of whom we didn't even know, collected our mail and left food for him outside our door every day. He made a list of people who left phone messages. He was astonished that we could know so many people, that they could have heard the news at all, that they could care so deeply. He opened piles of letters and saved them in a shopping bag, determined that one day I would read them. If I survived, I would need these records of my life as Rip Van Winkle to begin to cope with what had happened.

But being at home alone, even if it was on doctor's orders, made Jack desperate. For two nights my lovely Virgo ritualistically scrubbed and organized an already neat and clean apartment. He could not sleep, and a sponge made him feel like he was doing something. Finally, Jack had the good sense to move in with Juliana and Mark, down the street from MGH on Beacon Hill. He walked to the hospital early each morning, steeling himself against what he might find when he got there. Wind in the mountains, after all, can change in a second and bring on a storm.

His first day after the move, he passed a beggar on Charles Street who harassed him loudly. Jack switched to the other side of the street. The man kept yelling at him. Then Jack turned on his heel and marched right up to him.

"What's your name?"

"Marvin. What's it to you?"

"It means a lot to me if you know how to pray. Do you, Marvin? Do you know how to pray?"

Marvin looked at him through bleary eyes with the shock of the hunter who suddenly discovers that he is the hunted.

"Yes, sir, I can pray."

Jack moved in menacingly. He still has the swagger of the champion boxer he was at camp in Maine, a title he held until he became camp director and beating others to a pulp wasn't considered good leadership. Marvin cowered.

"You wouldn't lie to me, Marvin." A statement, not a question.

"No, sir. I'm a church-going man."

"Then here's five bucks and I want you to pray your brains out for my wife. I want you to stand here and pray all day. You bring her back to me, Marvin. You do it."

Jack was crying, and Marvin looked as though he'd seen a ghost. Right then he began to pray, loudly, and didn't stop. Every morning Marvin asked Jack how his missus was doing. He tried to wave away the money, but Jack would push it into his hand and sprint down the street.

Back in Great Barrington, Mary Kate tried to explain to four children under the age of eight what was going on. The questions were endless and often hilarious, like "Why did a heart attack Deborah?"

Each night they said grace before dinner and blew kisses to Boston. Everyone would blow in a different direction and a great fight would ensue. Wally was very intent on having the others blow in the direction he had determined was Boston because otherwise the kisses would get lost. One night Simon wanted to blow me some of his sloppy-Joe, his favorite meal. He was learning about sharing in kindergarten.

During the eight days that I was unconscious, Torch came two or three times a day to the waiting room, which now looked like a refugee camp. One day he reported incredulously that I was still moving, fighting to regain consciousness despite the heavy sedation. Jack was secretly thrilled with the report of my feistiness. After Torch left, he went in to see for himself. Ann saw him pause before my doorway and reach into his back pocket to pull out a small comb. He smoothed his hair neatly. She wanted to shake him, to tear him from his dream-world in which Sleeping Beauty would wake up and smile at him as on any other morning. She couldn't bear his pain, his delusion. Then she realized: Jack was actually coping well in the place he'd gone in his mind, and *she* was the one who needed to get a grip. They each had moments like this—swinging between clarity and disbelief, optimism and defeat. A comb through the hair was no different from her purchasing top-of-the-line running shoes to prevent my getting drop-foot, when old-fashioned Keds high-tops would have done the trick.

10

ON THE SIXTH DAY, they switched my medications to begin bringing me out of sedation and turned on the television in my room. In many hospitals this is standard procedure, a way of encouraging patients with familiar sounds. My sisters walked in to find *Wheel of Fortune* squawking. I was twitching. The nurse was puttering around doing useful things for me and didn't seem to notice.

"Deborah never watches television. I think she's bothered by this," Ann said in her most controlled and sweet voice.

"We put on the TV for most patients. It soothes them."

"Deborah hates television," Ann said with mounting anger—not just on my behalf but for any patient expected to awaken' peacefully to a game show. "Just look at her."

They switched off the TV. I relaxed a little and smiled.

Only one person at a time was allowed in my SICU room. Jack was usually at my side, holding my hand, talking to me, kissing my barely recognizable head—puffy with fluids and attached to a neck as thick as a tree trunk—leaving only to sleep for a few hours. On the seventh day, at 6 A.M., Callie woke suddenly from her vigil in the SICU waiting room with a premonition and asked permission to see me. As she entered the room, my eyelids fluttered a little. Though I was still unconscious, Callie sat slowly on the bed, barely able to contain her excitement, and gently told me the story of my last week yet another time, in case I was awake in there. I shook my head back and forth as if to say, "Can you believe this?!" A single tear dripped from one eye. Then Callie, my fellow early riser for the town swim team when we were kids, gave me an image I could grasp in case I could hear her.

"You are swimming in the lake, Deborah. Keep going," she said. "You are almost there—three-quarters of the way across. We're all waiting and cheering."

I have no memory of any of this, but I remember being in the lake, the velvety chill of clean water, and trying.

* * *

That afternoon, Marc came to the SICU waiting room camp and sat down, unable to hide his disappointment. In fact, the whole medical team was having difficulty maintaining their clinical distance—they were all deeply involved now. He began factually, as was his custom.

"We measure heart strength by ejection fraction, the percentage of blood expelled from the left ventricle with each heartbeat. The normal EF range is 50 to 70 percent. Michael Jordan's might be about 75 percent and, from what I hear of Deborah, hers might have been around 65 percent. Her EF prior to the operation was 8 percent . . ." He drifted off. Everyone knew what he meant.

Jack was not present, having gone back to our apartment with our friend Steven to sort mail and gather some things. In the room were my sisters, Juliana and her husband, Mark, and a friend of Jack's from work. Their eyes—every shade of blue, green, and brown—turned to black balls riveted on Marc.

"Deborah climbed from 8 to 15 percent immediately post-op. Our latest test shows that she is at 20 percent—a stunning occurrence, really, given the state she arrived in." He looked at the group to see if they were buying his enthusiasm. He had hoped to see a greater rise— to maybe 30 percent—because the biggest spike a patient experiences is in the first few weeks following surgery. After that, the EF usually levels off.

What the numbers meant was that I might come out of anesthesia significantly diminished. They couldn't hear Marc say that many people lead acceptable, though restricted, lives with EFs in the twenties. For them, there was only the likelihood that I would be a ghost, if I came back to them at all.

The mood in the room crashed. Marc decided to try another tack, reminding everyone that a significant portion of my heart muscle had been permanently damaged by the infarction in the first place, and that surgery had been performed not to return me to perfect health but to prevent further damage. No one fell for his pitch, though.

Shortly after Marc left, Jack and Steven bounded in, still thinking of my fluttering eyelids and filled with hope that I'd wake up tomorrow. Rebecca rose to relay the news in perfect detail, applying the youngest child's years of experience as a reporter when we called home to get news of one another. Jack froze, unable to speak, thinking the unthinkable: *Are you telling me that Deborah won't be the same?*

That evening, Jack and my sisters fled the hospital for the outside world. Steven left to pick up another friend, planning to meet Jack later at Rebecca's Restaurant on Charles Street. My sisters decided to give Jack some privacy and went their own way. After walking until they were tired, they chose the nearest restaurant and quickly had a couple of drinks. When the salad came, Ann found a big, black, unmistakable bug in the lettuce and looked helplessly at Leesa, tears pooling. Leesa marched to the bar, in charge.

"Look, my sister's in the hospital recovering from a double bypass and there is a bug in the salad." Leesa stood at the bar, intractable, glaring at the poor bartender, who struggled to put the two ideas together.

"We just can't handle it. Do you understand? A bug is unacceptable. There is a *bug* in the salad."

She burst into tears and returned to the table, spent. Then the laughter came. A bug in the salad. Only a bug in the salad!

In the meantime, Jack walked for a while in a daze, marveling that people he passed on the street couldn't see that his life had just shattered. He wandered into the Hampshire House, known as "The Cheers Bar," and ordered a martini. A blowsy woman plunked herself beside him and ordered a drink, chattering flirtatiously about the wedding she'd just left. Jack stared right through her, horrified by the thought that this could be his life, that his wife could actually die and he would be alone with no one to protect him from invasions like this. He paid for the drink, left it full to the brim on the bar, and walked to Rebecca's to wait on a stool beside the cashier. Steven had to lead Jack by the hand to their table; Jack hadn't even seen him enter, though he was staring fixedly at the door. Having dared optimism, Jack had plummeted to what he describes as his lowest point. The nightmare was not going away.

The next day my sisters, all in the fashion and design industry, practiced positive imagery: they discussed my new wardrobe. Jack sat in silence.

"She'll be the old Deborah in her favorite clothes—loose dresses to her ankles, not those horrible suits and pearls." Leesa, always specific in her dreams, imagined me in periwinkle.

During my stay in the SICU, Jack's body was either with me or in the waiting room, but all the while he was watching his own private movie. In it I was moving through my garden in a ratty old dress, carrying an overloaded weeding basket and wearing my big hat. At the mention of a *blue* dress, he woke up for a moment, encouraged that my sisters saw the film, too.

"Do you really see her wearing a dress?"

"Yes, Jack. It's blue." Leesa immediately sensed his despair and moved in close. Ann held his hands. I had blipped off his inner radar screen and he was panicking.

"Really?"

"Of course. She'll be wearing the soft, flowing clothes that she really likes, like the old days," Ann said.

"You're sure? I just can't see her anymore. I just can't see her wearing a dress and walking around anymore. Are you very sure?"

11

AS I COME TO THE SURFACE, I can feel his hand. He doesn't have a name yet, but I know this hand: it fits mine perfectly. I squeeze it three times. It is the magic squeeze that Mum taught us: three times means "I love you." She would deliver this private message when we were embarrassed or hurt, when we were introduced to a stranger who was old and scary, or when one of her girls was smeared with red lipstick at a dance recital. I taught it to my husband. Yes, that's whose hand it is, Jack's. (He collapses into someone's arms while the others take turns squeezing my hand to be sure he is not imagining it.) Now I am holding a different hand. I squeeze that one, too, just for the heck of it. There is a lot of screaming.

I open my eyes and everyone I love is at the foot of my bed. They are all double. Even my sister-in-law is here, so my brother must be, too. *Uh-oh, that means something's REALLY wrong.* They are smiling at me like fools, two smiles each. I grin back, reassured that a party is going on. It doesn't feel like a good grin, though. Something is in my mouth, but I smile to please them as best I can. I feel all warm. I can only see straight ahead, so I do not know that my husband is beside me, weeping. In fact, I've immediately forgotten that I'm married. I do not know that I am in a hospital.

Someone asks me if I would like to see Henri. *Oh, yes. Jack is my husband and he works with Henri. Where is Jack?* Henri comes close to my mouth. I find it odd, but I muster my best hostess skills anyway and smile.

"How nice of you to come, Henri!"

I am delighted to receive him at my party, but he is crying.

I have been unconscious for eight days and today is our eighth anniversary. Only Jack realizes this. We've made it.

I am on a red and green leather beanbag that I have not seen since horrid eighth-grade spin-the-bottle parties in knotty-pine basements. One leg is dangling uncomfortably off the beanbag. I try to pull my leg back to my body and discover something hard that I can push my foot against. I suddenly realize that I am choking. *I am choking.* I begin to hit the hard thing with my foot with all my might. *How did sneakers get back on my feet?*

I travel way back to a time when there were only two people in the world, making mud pies and pretend-cooking them on the stone fireplace in the backyard, and my mind calls *Callie, Callie.* From the waiting room down the hall, she feels my call and appears. I pantomime a pen and paper. She brings it to me and I scrawl CHOKING.

Callie turns accusingly to the nurse, pointing to the endotracheal tube connecting me to the respirator. "When are you taking this thing out?"

I look at her gratefully. After all these years and all the distances between us, Callie can still climb into my mind. We are still in the tree house together.

The nurse is unfazed. She assures Callie that the tube will come out soon.

54

* * *

I can vaguely see a nurse with I-Love-Lucy glasses who seems to have helped remove the tube as Callie promised me. I don't know yet that Doreen has been constantly at my side, even when duty did not require hovering. She told my appreciative sisters that her young daughter had been ill almost since birth. She had spent many days in the hospital wondering if her little girl would live or die, and she acted like it: quick, attentive, sensitive, calm.

Thank god that tube is out. I feel all slithery.

I am craving chicken broth. I can almost taste it: silken, richly seasoned, warm. I recall the chicken broth with tortellini and hot pepper flakes my friend Maria brought me years ago, which cured me of a cold, lost love, everything.

"We have some nice juice with ice for you here, Deborah," someone says to me loudly.

I don't like ice.

They want me to drink chilled things to take down the swelling in my throat, which is now larger than my head. For days I will continue to look like an inflated giraffe, but I don't know this. I don't know that my voice squeezes out of me in a whisper. Why are you all inches away from my face when I speak? I'm embarrassed because I feel a little dried drool in the corners of my mouth. I do not realize it is blood that continues to seep out, even though they wash me constantly.

I want chicken broth and I prevail. It is warm and savory, but I can still tell that it is from a can. I try to hide my disappointment. I would think they'd make really good chicken stock for someone who just came from NOTHING. I make a mental note to discuss this with the chef in this hotel. I'll teach her how to make it when I am stronger.

My bowels are moving oh-dear-do-something-fast, and a nurse swoops a bedpan beneath me with the flourish of a waiter pulling out a chair. The smell is vile. Everyone is so pleased, as though I am a baby. I find it especially interesting because my sisters have always squirmed with intense embarrassment at the mention of any bodily function, which made puberty a solitary affair for each of us. I like this new world.

Now Juliana is leaning close to my face. I grin up at her, in love. She says loudly to my nose, "Deb, we're taking Jack home with us now. He is very tired. He needs his rest, but he'll be back in the morning."

Oh, good. Jules is here. I am so happy for Jack to have a nice meal at their apartment. I whisper my instructions.

"Just be sure you make him a very large martini."

Everyone is suddenly whooping and clapping like I just hit the softball, finally, pitched gently to me in the front yard. Now where do I run?

Torch's biggest fear, after bringing me back to life, was that I would be brain-dead or at least brain-damaged. Had my brain been cut off from oxygen during the heart attack, and for how long? Torch had warned the family of this possibility and they waited for my first conversation to learn who I would be.

I had been a lover of words, a child who played with sentences. For me words were keys, each one holding the possibility of unlocking the truth. Yet my third sentence out of anesthesia had more meaning than anything I have ever written, ever said. For my doctors, it expressed reflection back in time, forward-looking vision, humor, recognition, the senses. I had hit the softball, all right, and it sailed past the swing set and into the woods, too far for anyone to stop it. I was still me. Martini.

12

TONIGHT I AM CROSS. Someone is playing music—awful music—way past bedtime. From the netherworld of the drugged, I see a nurse far, far away across a room that seems to me like a huge, jumbled freshman commons filled with oak furniture.

"Why am I in a room with all this spare furniture? Isn't there a real room available?"

My room was, in fact, slightly larger than a monk's cell, crowded with life-saving machines. The nurse explains that it is a perfectly nice room and that it's all they have.

"I can't believe MGH can't do better than this," I say, with cranky surrender and perhaps a bit haughtily.

The room is jammed with furniture that they have to move every time they lean over me, which is often. Why not just move it to storage? I don't see how they can function, but the lead nurse seems content. Perhaps the hospital is very crowded. I am lucky to have a room to myself, I guess. I drop the subject. Then I ask her about the music.

"What music?"

"The music piped into the hospital. Isn't it late for this? Aren't others trying to sleep?"

"I don't hear any music," she says. I think she is mad as a hatter; there is music everywhere, insistent, unrelenting.

When I open my eyes again I assume she has done her research on the music. Or has a day gone by? She reports that no music is being played anywhere that anyone can hear. I tell her about the room behind us where there is more oak freshman-commons furniture and where people are playing cards. I know they are playing cards, enjoying sandwiches and beer. I think the music is coming from doctors and nurses on their break playing a radio.

She comes up close to me and puts her hands on either side of my face. "There is no music, Deborah, and this is not a recreation room. You are hallucinating. It's the drugs. It's all in your head."

"But—"

"Would I lie to you? Would I?" Now she is cross. I must have been at her about this for quite a long time, but this is the first time I remember.

"No, you wouldn't lie to me; I know that," I say softly, cowed.

Meanwhile, my mind twirls out of my body like a genie and grins above me. *Great news! Hallucinations! If this is in your head, then you can change the channel!*

I think hard about Bach, conjuring up a few bars from a lovely cantata. It works and I feel smug with my new trick as the nurse gives me the first sponge bath that I can feel. I am a dead weight, but she is strong and turns me effortlessly. Or maybe there are four hands that I feel. My fresh cotton johnny smells so much better than the other one, drenched from the puddles on my bed. I am embarrassed to put her to this trouble. I go to sleep struggling to keep the Bach on and my body out of the puddles.

It bothered me for a long time that, in my journey back to full consciousness, I had criticized the chicken broth and the decor of my hospital room. But it's a good example of a phenomenon doctors and nurses know well: a stay in intensive care can unhinge the mind. The disturbance even has a name: ICU psychosis. It is being observed with increasing frequency as intensive care units proliferate in the United States. Something about the environment of the intensive care unit makes some patients already experiencing high levels of stress, debility, and pain lose their minds. Is it sensory deprivation? Or sensory overload from being tied to noisy machines day and night? Is it sleep deprivation and disruption of normal circadian rhythms? Whatever the cause, experts define it as "an acute brain syndrome involving impaired intellectual functioning which occurs in patients who are being treated within a critical care unit." And patients hallucinate sounds more often than sights, so I was right on track.

In a fascinating article on the subject that appeared in the *New York Times* in 1998, Dr. Sandeep Jauhar wrote that it is one manifestation of the more general phenomenon of delirium. Delirium, or acute brain failure, often has organic causes. Dehydration, infection, low blood oxygen, inadequate cardiac output, and drugs can all bring it on. I was pretty loaded with causes, both environmental and organic, but my condition was mild compared to some of my floormates.

I am floating in blue mist, a Picasso blue-period painting, inside a fish tank faintly glowing with cold, wobbly light. Mechanical things go*beep . . . beep . . . beep*, the submarine Muzak provided by this hotel. My body sloshes like the ocean, lulling me back to sleep though it is morning. Or *is* it morning in this watery, blue painting? I want to sleep. Why am I so tired if I am resting in bed in a nice hotel?

Lying in my watery pool just below the surface, I look up and see a man bending over me. First I see dimples. Then his eyes change from dots to curved slits, like the drawings of happy eyes in cartoons. Jack is standing behind him and introduces me.

"Deborah, this is your cardiologist, Dr. Marc Semigran."

The man is smiling at me. I love his eyes. I think but do not say, *Yes thank you very much it is nice to meet you but really I do not know what a cardiologist is and you are certainly not MINE.* My smile is a worm and I hope this Marc doesn't notice that I would rather be alone with Jack right now.

Now it is another blue morning, or perhaps it is the same one, or the one before. I am awakened by a deep booming male voice. I swim up to the top of the aquarium and see a frightening sight: a large man with shaggy hair and a droopy mustache. His voice is loud. I am irritated that he woke me up, now that I finally got to sleep. I can't sleep well in this hotel; they keep the lights on all the time.

Last night I thought I very nicely requested a change in the schedule, since I am young and I get the feeling that there are elderly people living here with me who don't need much sleep—why else would the lights be on all the time?

"Do you think I could be the first one you bathe at 9 P.M. instead of later? You see, I always go to sleep at nine and I'm up by six, in the office by seven-thirty. I would like to return to my routine." It is hard enough for me to be in a hotel unable to bathe myself; one would think they could be more flexible about timing.

The nurses sanely offered an explanation I could not follow and my request seemed to be denied. It was hard to tell. Night and day are all the same for me, as though I am adrift on a midnight sea when water and air have become the same element. But I didn't fuss further, since the young night nurses were nice and pretty and I wanted so badly for them to rub me with rough, clean, cotton cloths warm with soap so I could finally sleep.

And no sooner have I fallen asleep than it is morning again and I am awakened by a booming man leaning over me. I am afraid of him.

"Mrs. Heffernan, I am Dr. Torchiana, your surgeon." *What on earth do I have a surgeon for?* I do not smile for him.

"We have a very effective and aggressive recovery program here, and I want you to sit in a chair today." *Are you out of your mind? I am too tired. Perhaps if you would leave now so I can sleep.*

"And I note that you have not begun eating solids yet as we asked you to. No more broth and juice. Joanne will give you something more substantial."

He leaves and my nurse Joanne comes over to my head and puts her face close. "Joanne, who *was* that guy, anyway?"

I love Joanne. After the loud doctor is finally gone, she reclines the big chair so I can sleep in it. Then a male nurse lifts me up like a bride and gently positions me so I can eat. I can't help him at all; my right leg burns and I am limp as a wet noodle, ashamed. Exhausted.

I gag on the custard that Joanne brings me, a pale sweet puddle in a plastic cup. Then she tries Cream of Wheat. I eat a few bites because I am a good Girl Scout who learned on chilly mornings at Camp Green Erie that Cream of Wheat is nutritious. But this is solid and revolting. She offers Jell-O. I draw the line there and beg for soup.

Here now is a perfectly pea-green pea soup. But it tastes like pureed cardboard. Oh, how could they have ruined something that looks so lovely? I tell Joanne how to make pea soup, with a ham bone, garlic, and white wine. She is salivating, too. I pretend this is potage St. Germain and eat a few spoonfuls. So much for breakfast.

Jack, friends, and family were with me every day for the twelve days that I was in the SICU. Since I was hallucinating badly, I remember no one except the medical team, especially Joanne, who was tiny and blond with a little voice. High as a kite, I saw every handsome male medic as her potential husband. She indulged me and laughed at my meddling. She was my buddy. One day an elderly lady was yelling horrible, abusive things, protesting a procedure. Joanne was running between both rooms, trying to care for her and for me. Her pretty face was tense. I felt protective and asked her how she could handle a job where people were so mean to her. She looked at me with surprise.

"Oh, she's not mean. She's just scared. It's the drugs. They affect people in different ways."

Even in my druggy haze I began to understand that I was in expert, compassionate hands—hands that might change as I moved from one cardiac care team to the next, but whose standards were the same. I gave her a bouquet of flowers that arrived for me, forbidden goods in the SICU. I wanted so badly to pamper her, to bring her a cup of tea.

The young doctors doing their daily rounds were my early morning birdsong. Only the birds were crows, and the sounds they made were grim. They would arrive suddenly, with dark and somber faces. One of them seemed to be the leader and would bark questions at them in a monotone. He was handsome, tired, and stern. I thought he should lighten up, but no words came from my mouth—I hope. Besides, the other doctors didn't seem to notice his manner. I watched and listened.

"Mrs. Heffernan is doing remarkably well, considering her catastrophic first presentation."

Oh, dear, I bombed a presentation. It's only happened a few times in my career but always leaves me reeling with shame. I tried to focus on his compliment instead.

In general, medical vocabulary perplexed and amused me. At first I resented it. It seemed euphemistic, cowardly. I wanted the raw, cold, clinical facts. As I grew accustomed to this new language, however, I began to appreciate its precision. *Catastrophic first presentation, insults to the heart, irritated heart, cardiac event, invasive procedure*—these were actually vivid, unflinching descriptions of the truth. I could picture a cranky cartoon heart with arms and legs flailing inside my chest.

"Wow, what great sneakers!" No one has spoken like this to me in a long time. I do not know this voice. It is high and squeaky and delighted. I peer from my haze and see a large African American beauty strolling confidently into my room, her hair in braids.

"What sneakers?"

"Above your head on the shelf, honey. Boy, somebody must love you to buy you those sneakers."

She pulls them down from the shelf and shows me. They are hideous, stark white leather with high sides and lots of padding. They are also huge, so I explain to her that they could not possibly be mine.

"Oh, yes they are. Your sisters bought them for you."

Why would they buy me sneakers when I have a perfectly nice old pair at home? Maybe they're for walking out of the hospital. Leesa, our fashion maven, clearly had a hand in this. She probably convinced the others that my old running shoes weren't fancy enough. They are the last thing on earth I would wear. And don't they know my size? My feet are so skinny that I've walked right out of my shoes on the sidewalk.

I accept my visitor's praise politely and watch her move confidently about my room. She is happy and talks to me in a full, normal voice. I like her. She makes me feel like myself. Then she turns to me conspiratorially. "I have the same love with my husband that you have with yours. We hold hands all the time, like you do. Aren't we both lucky?" Oh yes.

"What are you doing, Deborah?" A nurse scurries in, prompted by blips from the central monitor.

As a matter of fact, I'm glad you came. I am having difficulty shifting to my side, my favorite position for sleeping with Jack, our arms wrapped around each other. I could use a little help. Another nurse appears, looking equally concerned. In the process of rearranging myself for when Jack comes to bed, I apparently pulled out a few of the million plugs in me. They find me tangled in wires and do not chastise me, just go with my insane request to make the bed ready for Jack. *Where is Jack? Why can't he come to bed with me?* I think there is room. The night nurses say no. They tuck pillows against my back so I can pretend he is there, and pillows in my front so he can be there, too. Then I am alone.

Sleep comes hard. The music in my head has changed. I can't get my Bach channel, only a Rachmaninoff concerto. At first it is pleasant, but then it goes into hysterical trills up and down the keyboard until I think I will scream. When I do sleep, I am disturbed by rapid-fire dreams, bursting like Roman candles. I do not remember them in the morning.

13

JOANNE IS BUSTLING ALL AROUND ME, much faster than usual. She seems a little flustered. Her voice trembles with excitement as she takes me through my morning ablutions. "What's all the fuss, Joanne?"

"We're moving you today!"

"That's nice," I reply, as indifferent as though she had said it's raining.

Being sedated makes you feel bland, like spongy white bread full of air. I greeted every bit of news flatly, grasping little of it. Marc said I began to ask questions about what happened immediately after coming out of sedation, though I seemed to absorb the answers like coins in a slot machine that never delivers. Good man, he didn't realize that was just the beginning of my questions. I was born asking, "Why?"

I kept passing out between answers. Minutes or a day would go by, and I would return to where I left off. I would forget everything that had been explained to me, often within seconds, and ask the same question again. My doctors and loved ones patiently repeated the story of my lost eight days, each time adding a little more information. Yet in spite of the tireless explanations, all I knew was that I was very sick. So when Joanne announced I was moving, I did not grasp what she meant: I was strong enough to leave intensive care and move to what's called the cardiac CCU (critical care unit) or Step-down, the eighth floor in the Ellison building, known to all as Ellison-8.

Bustling Joanne insists on bathing me for the second time this morning. Normally I love it, but I am a little achy and oh-so-tired. She looks tired, too.

"Oh, Joanne, don't bother doing this again. I'll be fine. My johnny's a little damp, but I don't mind."

"No, Deb, we really have to do this."

"But I don't mind, Joanne, and you have been so good to me. They can move me the way I am."

Joanne stands still beside my bed and leans on the mattress to support herself as she takes a deep breath.

"No, we really have to do this, Deborah," and she pauses, mustering courage, "because you smell." She giggles nervously and looks to see if she has hurt my feelings or gone too far in our casualness with each other.

So I haven't been imagining it! I was wondering who smelled like that! Even after my nightly baths I have been repulsed by the odor of my body as I try to sleep.

"Oh, dear. Do I smell all the time, Joanne? Has it been horrid for you?"

"Not at all. It's the drugs and it's normal. I just want you nice and fresh before we move you, or what would they think of me?" Anything for Joanne. Tired as I am, I submit to another drenched johnny being peeled from my body.

So, I smell. This new information does not slip out of my brain because I can smell me, too.

I am Cleopatra on her barge being wheeled out of the SICU: Everyone is smiling. I am sad to be leaving but pleased that Joanne is with me, escorting my barge just as Humphrey Bogart steered *The African Queen* through water teeming with crocodiles and leeches. The corridors feel as threatening.

The world is big and bright. I squint. Hallways glisten. People rush by. The ceiling is moving fast. I am dizzy with all the commotion of real life and the rocking gurney, which they seem to be pushing with amazing speed, negotiating the crowds. People stare at me. I smile back. All my tubes are with me, along with a big metal box called a defibrillator. I am in their hands.

A new nurse, Debbie, takes over for Joanne. *I had a feeling that's what this move meant. Why can't I still have Joanne?* I try to show my disappointment to the new nurse so that Joanne will stay. But Joanne quickly disappears, like a mother who rips a Band-Aid off before you can squawk. I am bland and submissive again.

Debbie's whole aura is one of warmth and competence, and I quickly transfer my devotion to her. Her voice is gentle and low. She looks tired, about-my-age tired. While I tumble happily into her kind, deep blue eyes, she gently pries the throat vacuum from my clenched fist. *No, no, no, no!* It has been my security blanket. I cannot breathe without this vile basting tube they've taught me to put in my mouth to suck out dead blood. I do not know why I have to do this, but I need to—otherwise, I choke. I have not yet mastered what the nurses call "productive coughing." Debbie soothes me by rubbing my back, but she does not let go of my vacuum cleaner.

"It's time to begin to do this on your own, Deborah. Besides, it's so dirty. You could get infected."

This scares me into surrender. *Why doesn't anybody let me do what I want to do anymore?*

Now Debbie sits down on the edge of my bed companionably and announces that it is time to order my dinner. I am overwhelmed. I don't want to eat, so how am I supposed to know what I want? All I really want is fruit juice and they keep making me eat other things, most of them pale and squishy. Debbie presents me with a one-sheet hospital menu that looks like a bad tie. It has tiny ovals all over it, with food listed beside the ovals. I cannot focus on it. So much, so much. I am exhausted from having been bathed twice today, followed by my barge ride. Thank heavens Ann is with me. She always seems to be there when I need her. I remember her voice, her touch. (In reality, everyone was there, not just Ann. But I was hallucinating and could only see one person at a time.)

"Ann, you choose. You know what I like to eat."

"Well, how about . . . the lasagna?" she says eagerly, choosing something uncontroversial. Ann's refrigerator contains fruit, crackers, and cheese.

But I cannot imagine eating. Certainly not something as heavy as lasagna. She reads aloud the other selections. I imagine instead a lighter meal of pasta cooked al dente and tossed with good olive oil, garlic, and flat parsley. Now that would be nice. The thought of drinking wine with it revolts me, though. That's probably why wine is not on the menu.

Debbie takes the menu from Ann and offers it to me tentatively, as though it's a gift she's unsure of.

"No, let her decide. She knows what she likes to eat."

In the with-it part of my brain I know that she is a pro: this is to be my first step toward independence. *Oh, yes, I remember now. My job used to be helping adults learn new skills.* Debbie now has my professional admiration. *OK, I get it. I get it.*

Lasagna it is.

At bedtime, as I settle back into my heavenly, hospital-scratchy pillows, I ask Debbie about the beautiful woman's picture on the ceiling above my bed in every room. I keep meaning to ask someone about it. She looks like Boston's notorious turn-of-the-century patron of the arts Isabella Stewart Gardner as she was painted by Zoran, bathed in light.

"Was Mrs. Gardner the hospital benefactress?"

"Oh, I don't know," Debbie says slowly as she looks up at the ceiling light, giving my question serious consideration to make me feel like I am having a normal conversation. "People see different things in that picture."

My Isabella was actually a high-intensity light that was flicked on in emergencies, when the doctors needed maximum visibility. But I believed it was my angel. She went with me to all three rooms at the hotel. Even when I was lucid, I still saw her as an angel. My Isabella.

I hate the night, but I didn't used to. Before I checked into this hotel it was my most treasured time of the day, when I crawled beneath the sheets with Jack, put my head on his shoulder, my nose in his fuzzy chest, and drifted off to a lovely sleep. Now every part of my body aches. I am only marginally comfortable sleeping on my back, a foreign and awkward position. The top of the bed is elevated slightly, the bottom bent into a sort of hillock for my knees. I pretend it is my hammock under the pines. I think so hard about this on my first night on Ellison-8 that I am actually there, swaying in the breeze with lake sounds in the air instead of the beeping of machines. I want so badly to sleep on my side but my chest aches, threatening to fold in two. I think about every part of my body and ask it to relax, to let go. I find tension even in my knees and they obey. Without yoga training I would not be able to do this. What is my yoga teacher, Zoe, thinking now? Did anyone call her? Where is my car?

As I finally drift off to sleep, the music starts. The Rachmaninoff trills are a nightmare, filling my head until it explodes. Then I hear horses' hooves on scree. I see them struggle to descend a sun-scorched slope. The music is a high-pitched whistle. Then I realize it is the theme song from *The Good, the Bad, and the Ugly*. I do not remember ever seeing this film or hearing the music before.

I am in a sweat. Someone changes me again. Here comes *Porgy and Bess*! I listen to the entire score, including the spoken parts between the songs. I haven't listened to all of *Porgy and Bess* since I was a teenager but, incredibly, I know every note. A night nurse comes to check on me again. I ask her if she can hear *Porgy and Bess*, just to test the hallucination.

"What's *Porgy and Bess?*" she asks. Oh, well. I didn't know what a "cardiac event" was before, either.

The room is dark and quiet. I open my eyes and see no difference. Then the voice comes to me again. It is a lovely, lilting bass voice. It is coming from a glowing green hospital shirt suspended in the air above me. The shirt is wide at the shoulders and narrow at the waist.

"My name is Eric, De-bo-rah, and it's time to draw your blood."

"Nice to meet you, Ellie," I whisper sleepily. "You have to take it again so soon?"

"I'm sorry De-bo-rah. You must be tired of this—three times a night. I'll make it quick. Then I'll turn you. I'll be coming in to turn you a few times tonight."

The green shirt does the blood work. It is a vaguely familiar sensation and I think they have done this to me before. I do not realize that so much blood has been taken from and given to me that until recently a shunt had been in my neck. Then the green shirt lifts me and I feel that he has arms. Big strong arms, which must be why the shoulders are so big in the shirt. He moves me like a father picks up a child and I feel so happy, so protected by this prince, saved from the dragons.

"Where are you from, Ellie?"

"I am from Costa Rica."

"Oh, yes. I know where that island is."

He lets it go.

The next morning I am embarrassed at my gaffe; I certainly know that Costa Rica is not an island. I do not know, however, that it is a big deal to recognize a mistake, any mistake—that my brain is working, very well. I try to send an apology to the green shirt, but no one knows a male night nurse named Ellie.

"Gooood mornnning!"

Janice breezes in, all business, deposits my breakfast tray, and glides out. An aide follows up by placing the tray in front of me on the moving table and cranking up my bed. Then she lifts the cover off my food and leaves.

I stare at scrambled eggs and sausage, buttered toast, juice, cereal, coffee. I sit for the longest time trying to figure out what I am supposed to do with this. I am going to retch. Then a nurse comes in and whisks it away in disbelief.

"Good thing you got the wrong tray and not someone else on this floor. They would have eaten it!"

Janice returns, both apologetic and formidable. "Well, you didn't order breakfast, so we sent you the standard."

Standard?. Have I imagined this heart attack after all?

I am starving and at her mercy. I beg her to find something else. To Janice, I am lucid. She has no idea that this is my first morning in Step-down, my first time managing my own needs because until now a personal nurse has done everything for me. I remember the shock of first grade.

Janice is practical. So many people to feed, so fast. She returns with my request: yogurt, fruit, and juice. She makes it clear that it is not easy to get food after the initial rounds are completed. I explain my confusion and she softens. She sits on the edge of the bed and helps me open the yogurt.

"Okay, here is the system." She hands me a menu like the one Debbie filled out for me last night. "Every morning this will be delivered to your room and you'll order lunch, dinner, and breakfast for the next day. It's easy, all fill-in-the-dots." She smiles, pats my hand, and disappears.

Easy, yes. I try to pick up a pencil. I cannot do it. I try again. My fingers will not close around this implement I have used to write stories and draw pictures ever since I wore puffy skirts and ankle socks at birthday parties. I draw on last night's practice: I had eaten a few bites of the lasagna Ann cut up for me by using my fork only, stabbing my food. I had not counted on pencils as the next challenge. I take all morning filling in the dots and am exhausted by the time Janice returns to collect my order. She finishes it for me.

My first day on the floor I had a nurse who made me despair of human kindness. After my breakfast, she put me in a chair and did not give me the buzzer, a hand-held button that signals the front desk for help if you press it. And I didn't know to ask for it because I didn't realize that it existed. The nurse left me in my chair for what felt like hours but was probably only one. I had no voice with which to call her, no strength to adjust the position of my body, which was sinking painfully in the chair. Helplessly, I watched her talking and laughing at the main desk; like a surly waitress, she seemed to willfully ignore my faint waves. Not once did she look my way, although acute cases are always given rooms near the main desk precisely so they can be watched constantly. I was so tired and achy that tears begin to seep from my eyes. I resented her neglect. My anger rose and rose, and I knew that this was not a good feeling for someone recovering from open-heart surgery. Where was Debbie? Joanne? Jack?

And then it hit me. This is what it feels like to be old or paralyzed, a prisoner of your body—a nonperson for anyone who is healthy. It was the first time I had experienced being ill in the land of the callously well. And a cardiac nurse was my initiator.

I was pleased to hear that she resigned soon after that. She was actually a good nurse who had been at it for too many years and had burned out. I could tell.

"No, please don't! Don't take out my catheter! I love the catheter." *Whatever will I do if this thing is removed?*

I am desperate about this next change. I want to go back to the SICU, where everyone was nice. First my throat vacuum, now the catheter. I have been drinking cranberry juice purposefully so there would be no infection. Next, they'll probably expect me to go to the bathroom on my own.

They do.

They crank my bed so I am sitting upright. Debbie supports my back while an aide lifts my legs over the side. There is that searing burn again. My johnny rides high on my thighs and I look down at my legs and squeal.

"What happened to me? Look at my leg!" The skin on my right thigh near my groin is a brilliant purple, the stain as big as a football. There is also a violent red gash, wrinkled like seersucker, running along the inside of the thigh, from my knee to my crotch. It is stapled together. *Without those staples, would it flap open?*

At this moment, Torch ambles in with his rounds board and soda.

"Good for you, Deborah. You're up."

"Torch, tell me about this," I demand, pointing to my purple, stapled thigh, the most horrid thing I have seen in my life.

"Oh. Sorry about the staples. We were in a bit of a hurry."

"In a hurry? For what?"

He sits slowly on a chair and speaks softly. "That's where we took the vein from, Deborah. For the bypass." I cock my head and so he tells me again, "You've had open-heart surgery and a double bypass. The leg is a good place to get the extra vein from."

Inside my body I am still as death. I've been told this before, I think. I can't believe someone cut my leg open. Certainly not Torch.

I try to cover the lurid railroad track with my johnny. I think I am about to vomit, but it subsides. Torch is filling me in kindly, directly. I barely listen. I look at him and I feel suddenly calm. He is my hero.

Two people assist me. It takes quite a while for me to stand. We wait for the dizziness to subside from my steady diet of medicine. They tell me never again to bolt up from a sitting position. I must stand, pause, then move slowly. *As if I could stand! As if I could run! As if I could move with my own steps, my own spirited steps!* Right now, the windows are sealed, yet I am swaying in the breeze. I try to put one foot forward and nearly collapse. This is the way we make it to the bathroom. It takes an eternity, and I really have to pee. I've learned that they have me on diuretics to keep me peeing all the time. *Who needs diuretics? Not me. I am a human river. Waste of a good drug.* A third person trails us with my IV trolley. We all go into the bathroom. Good thing I'm not shy or proud.

It is hard to ease up onto the toilet, built high for wheelchair users. The edge of the seat sticks to my legs and blocks the circulation. I ask for a stool to put under my feet. My right leg rips with pain. I urinate all by myself for the first time in almost two weeks. *Now isn't that just great.* I collapse back into bed. That's it for activity this morning. What a busy day!

14

WHEN THEY MOVED ME IN, my room was empty and I got the bed near the window. It looks out on a brick wall, but the light is more lovely than anything I have ever seen. It dances, it glows, it softens, it fades to gray mist and then navy blue. I watch it, enjoying every minute as the drugs wear off.

Suddenly an elderly woman is in the next bed. I don't know how she got there. Jack pulls the curtains to separate us, but I have seen enough. She is very frail, a little bag of bones well into her eighties. They call her "the pro"; this is her second bypass.

I hate her.

I will not attempt small talk across the curtain wall. I will pretend to be alone with the light. What on earth am I doing in a hospital bed, unable to walk, sharing a room with a heart patient, a woman twice my age? I am not ready for my new peer group. Besides, I am just learning how to cough "productively" and it is disgusting, even more so now that someone else can hear.

My new nurse-for-the-day quickly assesses the situation.

"We're outa here," Denise says as introduction, telling my husband and sisters to gather my things while she readies the gurney and IV trolleys. "One of my patients just checked out of 8-36. It's only got one bed and it's yours."

All that's missing are balloons and a band. We're giddy. We are running from the Andersons' apple orchard having stolen some wormy macs—the same thrill, the same hilarity. We race to claim the new room before anyone else can.

The privacy saved my life. Soon Ellison 8-36 filled with flowers. It was my garden. I pretended I was digging sweet compost into my own sour earth, continuing its transformation under the cathedral pines. Spring was in my room while outside it was still gray and cold. I kept the temperature chilly to pretend it was fresh air and piled on the blankets. The doctors, nurses, and aides lingered in my cool, fragrant garden. My window had a view of the Charles River, but I had to sit in a chair to see it. This forced me out of bed and retrained the muscles of my back. Fifteen minutes in my chair left me exhausted and achy beyond words.

From my chair I watched life go on, incongruously. Boats slowly purred along the Charles, filled with tourists. Slender cormorants dove for unsuspecting fish. Roller skaters whizzed by. Sailboats left zigzagging wakes. Sinewy, tanned mothers ran, pushing babies in jogging strollers. I could not imagine moving with their oblivious ease. It was marvelous, this pulsating life and its obliviousness.

At other times, nothing was amusing and I simply got good and pissed off.

I am sitting in my chair eating breakfast, watching the world outside. I have not yet mastered stabbing pieces of fruit with a fork. Slippery devils. Usually, it takes me most of the morning to move one piece to my mouth. The rest of the morning I spend chewing it—my tongue still so swollen and numb from the intubation that it is useless. Then it's time for a nap.

I have just speared a piece of melon when a stocky man with a trim brown beard appears. He looks a little like Hemingway at his finest. Green eyes twinkle at me above the beard. He moves a chair right over to me, takes my hand, and looks into my eyes like a lover.

I get the feeling we've met before, and ask shyly, "Are you another person who knows my body better than I know it?"

"Yes, I suppose I do," he chuckles. "Dr. Greg Koski, your anesthesiologist during surgery. I wanted to wait until the lady was more herself before I visited."

I vaguely remember Jack telling me that I was kicking and that they had to strap me down. I had pulled at the straps, straining as though my life depended on escape. I wish I could have been more cooperative.

"Sorry. I understand I really fought you and your team."

"Fought us! Far from it. You were fighting for your life. We'd never seen anything like it. You inspired us. Your spirit told us you were staying right here. You arrived nearly dead and kicking, and we gave you enough drugs to put down a horse. But you still kicked through. I had to meet the lady who belongs to that spirit."

What is the spirit? Does it ever reveal itself fully unless we are pressed to the extreme? You can actually see some people summon it, like Olympic athletes preparing to sail over the high jump or pumping to the finish line. Others reveal it in their unbridled laughter, in eyes filled with tears of compassion. But you can see the spirit most vividly in the eyes of the dying, telling punctuation at the end of a life.

My husband knows what it is like to be distilled to pure spirit. The 1978 leader of one of the first American teams to summit Aconcagua, the highest mountain outside of the Himalayas, Jack was hit with the undiscriminating altitude sickness pulmonary edema. He was immediately lowered from 21,000 to 12,000 feet and pumped full of medicine and fluids. A climber was assigned to stay with Jack, a plan they had all agreed to should something like this happen to any member of the team. Jack's best friend Morrie took over as expedition leader as they made their way to the summit.

Once alone with Jack, the climber said he was going to look for more water and, unaccountably, didn't return for days. As deliriously sick as Jack was, he knew he couldn't survive long at that altitude without more fluids and someone caring for him. He tried to crawl down a steep scree slope 4,000 feet above a rushing glacial river, the same river he saw in the linoleum floor that separated us at Mount Auburn Hospital. A few minutes into his descent, he knew he did not have the physical strength and crawled back to slowly drown to death in his own fluids, betrayed by his body and a friend, kept alive only by his spirit. Jack lasted three days under the glaring sun, when he should have been dead in one. Just as I had kicked the team of anesthesiologists, Jack raised his jackknife to the team of Spanish climbers who saved his life; in his hallucinations he thought they were pirates. Like me, he could count only on his spirit, and it did not let him down.

I want to tell Dr. Greg this, but I do not have the breath. I want him to know that my spirit is not mine alone, that I would never abandon Jack on a scorched scree slope without a hell of a fight. But he already knows this because true healers understand that the body does not work alone. After all, he was the doctor who had urged my family to kiss my drugged body on its trip to the operating room, sending me off with love whose touch I might remember deep below the sedation.

I see Wendy's belly first. She is my new nurse and eight months pregnant. She waddles in with the sure gait of pregnant women who are cherished and happy. She beams at me and I rise up like a flower.

"How about a real sponge bath?"

Oh love at first sight! Oh bliss! Oh rapture! Sing songs to Wendy! She helps me out of bed and I show off my new trick: shuffling to the bathroom by myself while leaning on the IV trolley. She sits me down on a little bench and I slowly brush my teeth and spit into the sink. While my tongue is still too swollen to cooperate much, clean teeth are grand, awkward dribbles and all. We stand me up and untangle me from my damp johnny and IV lines. She rinses a fresh white washcloth in baby soap for me to use all by myself.

But I am stunned by what I see in the mirror. The band stops playing. The carousel jerks to a stop.

My hair is as wild as that of the schizophrenic woman I see walking along the Charles River digging in trash barrels. My face is pale as the pages of a book, my dark blue eyes, sunken black holes. My skin sags. I look fragile. I look sick. *Who is that?* I stare for a long time. Then my eyes travel south.

"*Wendy, what is wrong with my chest?* Look at it!" I gasp, thinking she will be surprised.

My chest has a shrieking red scar starting at my clavicle and traveling to my stomach. It sticks up like a mountain ridge. My neck bears the scar of the shunt. My bony shoulders cave in and won't lie back where they used to. On my belly are two marks about an inch long, as though someone stuck a knife in there. Then my eye travels to yesterday's news: my pubic hair is gone and my groin and upper right thigh are an enormous field of reddish purple. There are the staples all the way to my knee. I grip the sink and stare. This is not my body. I look into my eyes, and my spirit is hiding from me.

Wendy gently places me back on the bathroom stool and whispers, holding my eyes. "You've had open-heart surgery, Deb. It means that they open your chest to operate."

Could Torch have done this to me? I had to see it to believe it.

Later that morning, Jack arrives for lunch, carrying his paper bag. I turn to him abruptly from my chair, where I've been staring out the window, deep in thought. I am beginning to grasp what happened to me, what my family has been going through for weeks.

"Jack, do you think it was the crème brûlée?"

Knowing exactly what I am talking about, Jack kisses my forehead and perches on the edge of my bed, lunch bag rustling.

"No, love, but they did find some green sludge in your heart."

I try to sit up a bit, to be a good and alert pupil because he is clearly going to give me some new information about the chest I saw this morning, rising like the Rockies at dawn after a long drive.

"And the sludge clogged my heart?"

He nods solemnly.

"So, what was it?"

"The fiddleheads you ate."

People who undergo planned surgery are usually well prepared. Emergency open-heart surgery on someone who does not have cardiovascular disease is another thing entirely. Seeing myself was a shock, no matter how many times people told me what had happened. During the first three months after surgery, I relentlessly asked questions. The questions were desperate reflexes—like a foot twitching on a corpse. The answers were mere pieces to the puzzle, not the whole. The whole was beyond my comprehension.

It was inconceivable to me that Torch had sawed me open, then inserted a steel spreader and cranked its gears apart until my ribs opened enough for him to reach inside my chest. It was inconceivable that I had been a slab of meat whose heart Torch had held in those big, beautiful hands—hands that mesmerized me as he talked, that felt my ankles for swelling with warmth and gentleness. I felt like a child who's just been told that storks do not deliver babies. The reality was revolting.

At night I would think about my new life in the hospital. Try as I might to shut these thoughts out—to bring back even the dreaded Rachmaninoff, which had by now ceased—I would review every detail since May 12 in out-of-sequence flashes. Then, just as I was finally sleeping, a night nurse would appear to take blood or weigh me. Or I would suddenly feel a hot bullet shooting through my urethra and have to buzz frantically for someone to escort me to the toilet. Or the bell on the IV trolley would go *ding-dong ding-dong* until a nurse came to replace one of the empty bags with a new one.

Now I knew why, when I turned in bed, my chest felt like it could fold in two, why my right leg burned. My body was a wreck. I was reduced to being thrilled with a sponge bath or my recent mastery of the food order form. Jack brought me all the *New Yorkers* I had missed, which I devoured despite my wooziness. Friends instinctively knew my hunger and sent me piles of books to bring me back. Language was all I had left of who I had been.

The cleaning staff—shy, graceful women from Haiti, their hair in tiny braids or French twists—would enter my room to tidy, silent as moths. One day I could not think of the English word for what I needed and switched to French, mixed with a little German from the time when I had taught school in Switzerland. My Haitian savior flashed a huge smile and spoke with me in her beautiful singsong French until we figured out what I was trying to say in English. She asked me if I was Parisian. Nothing like Parisian schoolgirl French to get you by in a pinch. Unthinkingly, I had reached back into the landscape of my former life and found French limping about. I did not realize that this was significant at the time. I was simply pleased and a little vain.

The few French and German words I had uttered were another link to who I had been, evoking happiness. I began to calm myself by remembering a specific brilliant day in the Hasliberg of Switzerland, when I had gone for a hike into the Alps. In my mind the air was once again deliciously dry, thin, and fresh, the dirt path densely packed from centuries of use, my feet light and sturdy in boots that gripped my ankles. A herd of mountain goats followed me the whole day, stopping when I stopped, clamoring behind me when I moved on. I remembered the pure happiness of being twenty-three and seeing all of life ahead as a beautiful path up and down mountains. I reached for that again.

15

WENDY AND I SHUFFLE FAST into the room across the hall, which is actually one big shower. She warns me sternly to be quiet, that our morning's activity is taking place a little sooner than the doctors would like. I am to bend over on my stool and hold several thick towels to my chest which may not get wet. I agree. Anything for Wendy. Anything for a shampoo.

She presses her big belly against my shoulder and scrubs. Soap in the eyes. Who cares? Water and soap everywhere. We are giggling uncontrollably. Everyone on the floor can hear us—so much for the secret hair wash. Nothing has ever felt so divine.

We talk like girlfriends. In her swollen, tight belly is Wendy's first child. Wendy's mother is dying of cancer and she drives to western Massachusetts every week to be with her. She is not pleased with the care her mom is getting. Her parents are divorced, and her dad lives on Beacon Hill with his second wife. He's a workaholic consultant.

"Is that how you worked, too?" she asks me.

I don't want to think about that right now.

Wendy is twenty-eight, the same age as Jack's children. As I ask her more about herself, she comes into focus as someone with a life beyond the hospital, and I am in awe that she has any energy left for me, for all of us on the floor.

Gradually, I've been asking more and more questions of my caretakers and they are becoming multidimensional. Debbie is studying to be a nurse practitioner and recently had her third child; Torch's first child, a daughter who fits into his hand, has just been born; Marc's wife is also a cardiologist and they have two young daughters; Stan, Torch's PA (physician's assistant), runs the Boston Marathon every year in a Groucho Marx mask; Eric (my Ellie) has five children and the oldest is going to medical school. Through my slowly aroused interest in their lives, I reach for my place in life again, shifting my focus from the staples on my leg to the world beyond my epidermis. And this world is big; at least six countries, including Pakistan, are represented among my caregivers.

In gaining strength, I move tentatively out of my cave and into the light and air. But it is a different world. As my body pisses, sweats, and defecates the morphine out of me, I find my abruptly changed, newly uncomfortable world horrifying, yet more and more interesting.

Perhaps it is interesting because for the first time in my life I am in a position to observe everything with responsibility for no one but myself. I can watch and listen endlessly because I am too weak to do otherwise, and because my only real job is to heal myself. Later—in the same way that the lives of my immediate caretakers came slowly into view—I will think about the insurance that supports us (to the tune of more than $250,000 for my hospitalization alone) and how desperate others in my situation would be without it. Given how political I've been my whole life, it's a sign of how sick I am that I can't give the plight of others a single thought. All compassion has been sent on vacation. It is as though I were following the instructions given by flight attendants before takeoff: "In the event of an emergency, place the yellow cup over your nose and mouth before helping another person."

One morning, Juliana's husband, Mark, catches me crying. I spend days crying. The tears slip out with alarming ease, inspired by everything and nothing in particular, like water seeping from a lake overflowing with snowmelt. They flow over my granola, into teacups and conversations, onto my pillows and books. They come and go, but are always there like breezes. No one makes me feel self-conscious about them; we talk around my crying jags as though they are just another friend who has joined the conversation. My tears are partly induced by the drugs, but mainly by the dawning realization that life has changed irrevocably.

On his way to the hospital, Mark had passed Jack's friend the churchgoer, harassing people for change. He turned abruptly and startled the poor fellow, demanding, "Are you Marvin?"

"Yes," the man said tentatively, eyes darting.

"Well, that lady you've been praying for? She lived! You did it!"

Mark shoved twenty dollars into his pocket. Marvin's jaw dropped, then sewed itself right back up into a wide smile.

My tears turn to laughter. Then Mark pulls from a brown bag a paper mâché mask with eyes sculpted like flowers and an elastic band to go around my head for "one of those days," he says. I will wear it often when I need other people's laughter to trigger my own.

My sisters have given me a beautiful journal, hoping that I can put my tears into words. I am so delighted with this thoughtful gesture that I haven't been able to tell them that it is impossible for me to reflect, not just yet. Coping takes all my imagination. I use the notebook to record questions that I save for visits from my doctors and nurses. I cannot process information yet, but I can organize it.

The crow doctors from my SICU days swoop into my room at dawn. Each day they are cheerier, morphing into penguins. It must be my flowers. The handsome, cranky leader, Dr. Tom MacGillivray, even jokes with them. Then he summarizes the visit while the interns nod and scribble notes rapidly.

"All right, guys. What does all this mean?" I ask, flattening erudition. I am upright in bed, straining to apply my new medical vocabulary, but they are always ahead of me. I have my journal ready to record what they say and any questions I might want to save for Marc and Torch.

Tom grins at me. "It's time to report to our alert one. It means you're doing all right. You're doing amazingly all right."

"Tom, you were so grim in my room in the SICU. I thought you were mean. But you're really so nice!"

Laughter and blushes. They no longer look like doctors. They jab each other playfully. They are any gang of friends. Tension evaporates from Tom's face. Then he switches back to his professional role and smiles wanly.

"To tell you the truth, Deb, I can't help matching my demeanor to how serious the patient is. You were one sick puppy when we first met. I'm the chief resident in cardiac surgery and was the assisting surgeon for you. I worked with Torch."

We look at each other, and for me no one else is there. *So, you have seen my heart, too. You may have cracked my chest and split my sternum with an electric saw. Or did you remove the vein from my leg?*

Well.

Well, I looked forward to Tom's smile every morning. As long as there was mirth, I was fine.

One day, about a week after I had come out of sedation, Jack came to the hospital with two shopping bags of mail. Had he brought me this any sooner, I would not have grasped the enormity of what I'd been through. I went through the mail slowly, barely able to see for the tears.

There were pictures of newborn babies. Drawings from children— my nephew Chris's school photo stuck right in the middle of his in case I'd forgotten what he looked like. One, two, three notes from some people, surpassed only by Jack's cousins Joan and Agnes, who seemed to have written daily. Words of encouragement, words reminding me who I was. Words describing spring unfolding in gardens. The photo of our Maine neighbors holding the big GET WELL sign across our muddy driveway. I opened the small box of magic things from our land they had sent for me to smell—lake water, reindeer moss, spruce cones, dirt. Perri had painted beautiful watercolor postcards of famil- iar Maine spring landscapes. There was Bob's wooden medicine spoon in the shape of a snake. Misty had sent perfumed cream made with healing herbs that I saved for when the doctors would allow me to use it on my dry, cracked legs. And Lucia had photographed my tulips, knowing that I would hear their call.

It took me days to read through the two bags, and more kept coming. I had a telephone, but I kept it unplugged unless I needed to call out. Exhausted, I needed to reserve all my breath, like oxygen in a tank. Instead, I sat in my chair and looked out at the Charles, reading my letters as carefully as a history book.

A friend once told me about his memories of almost dying on an operating table, floating above his body and looking down at himself. This never happened to me. I know that I never left my body, never left this earth. I stayed in my sunny chipmunk's den, warm and happy. And I remember no pain. The bags of letters explained my cozy feelings as I broke the surface of the drugs: I'd been surrounded with love, near and far, just as the doctors had prescribed as they rolled my unconscious body into the OR elevator.

16

KEITH BOUNDS INTO THE ROOM, radiating cheer and robust health with his sandy-haired good looks and athlete's body. This is exactly how a physical therapist should look.

"So, ready to go for a walk?"

There is no one else in the room, so he must be talking to me, and I can tell he means a walk beyond the bathroom. I am terrified and thrilled. We take my IV trolley with us and I lean on it. A nurse supports me on one side and Keith supports me on the other. Even if I had been able to walk normally, I think I would have dragged my feet just to make the moment last. It is my first real walk in weeks.

I am seeing Ellison-8 for the first time without hallucinations. The floors are shiny and quiet. Nurses laugh at the main station at the end of the hall. Keith walks happily into the polish and fluorescent lights as though we are in a park. I shuffle beside him. He begins to lead me around the cardiac care unit, which is laid out in a loop.

There are pictures on the wall, gifts from the grateful. I pause and rest a lot, once in front of a print of a skier pounding through the woods on back-country skis. I stare. *Who am I now?* To remind me, Jack had brought in a picture taken just this last February on Mount Washington during the family's annual winter climb. I was helping his daughter Brenda put on her crampons. Now I am clinging to an IV trolley for dear life. It depresses me. I want my body back. I want to walk with wings on my feet like Keith, but today I have to turn back only halfway around the loop. I am spent.

Each day, someone from physical therapy came to take me through the paces. I did exercises in bed like flexing my feet and lifting my knees. It would exhaust me. Then we'd go out on the floor again. Gradually I did the whole loop—and eventually I could do it without leaning on the IV trolley; my therapist pal would push it. They assigned me three loops a day. I was *cruising*. And then some days I was just too tired; my blood pressure would drop again and they would ground me.

One day I was showing off for Keith. "Look, I can walk all by myself if you push the trolley."

We tooled around the loop in no time. I was flying with pride.

"That's very good, Mrs. Heffernan. Tomorrow we'll try lifting our feet."

I was crushed. I looked at my feet as if they had betrayed me. After a couple of more days I had the feet down. No more mincing shuffle for me.

"That's really good, Mrs. Heffernan," Keith praised. "Now tomorrow, we'll try swinging our arms."

Eventually I got so that I could walk *and* look around. Doing two things at the same time was yet another cause for celebration. But what I saw was not good: room after room of pasty-faced, overweight people, many with the yellow skin of smokers, all over sixty, most of them men. I had been such a good girl, honoring my body. My one sin had been a vodka martini before dinner, and the doctors joked that had they known I was so squeaky clean, they would have prescribed it. My grief turned to resentment, and resentment became anger. Some of my fellow patients had probably had heart disease or diabetes since birth, but I wasn't making distinctions; I was just mad. In my nasty mood, these anonymous lumps in bed had done conscious damage to their bodies and then expected MGH to pick up the pieces of their wrecks.

One of the nurses told me how depressing it was when former patients visit in crisp civilian clothes reeking of cigarette smoke. Just thinking about it made me want to scream at my floormates. It was a good thing I couldn't yet walk, look, and talk at the same time.

I am blinking myself awake in the gray light of early morning. Torch appears in my room ahead of the residents today. He has come straight from the OR, his mask dangling from his neck, his footsteps muffled in paper booties.

"You look tired, Torch. Have you been up all night?"

"Yeah, a heart transplant." He states his business as matter-of-factly as a lawyer would say "a deposition."

"How did it go?" I ask, trying to pretend his work is not beyond casual inquiry. I see the fatigue in Torch's shoulders, the driven eyes. I know he is preposterously here without skipping a beat, to begin his rounds, to see me and hear how I am. But for the moment I want to make him my patient. He relaxes, but only a little.

"Not that well, Deborah. I don't think it's going to take. I don't feel good about it. Now, how are you? Loosen that thing a bit so I can check the scar."

He helps me untie my johnny and squints at my zipper (hospital jargon for the chest incision), completely absorbed. I revel in Torch's attention, his polite examination.

"Nice job, Torch," he says out loud to himself as he gets up to leave, admiring the healing that only he can see. His eyes smile a little.

I feel foolish for taking his time. *I'm fine! Go save another life!* But maybe this visit to one of his successes has given Torch calm and focus. I do not realize that in his eyes I am still acute. Instead, I pour my prayers into that anonymous body with the new heart, lying inert in the SICU. I remember the light and sounds that he does not yet know.

My bond with Torch was and still is especially deep. Does the body instinctively know when its life has been saved and by whom? Since he had touched and healed my physical heart, my spiritual heart simply fell in love—just as a recently hatched gosling attaches itself to the first face it sees, whether it is a goose or a human being. No matter how bad I felt on Ellison-8, I would always rise like a sparkling wave for Torch, my torch of light.

He has the same impact on everyone, I've come to realize. At his approach, our friends' and family's body language was a mixture of standing at attention and rushing in for a cuddle. The nurses love him because he respects them when other surgeons can behave petulantly. And his dedication extends beyond MGH: he once talked Marc Semigran and a whole surgical team into spending Thanksgiving in China, operating and teaching continuously for three jet-lagged days before returning to Boston. It's hard to refuse him.

Ann is with me this afternoon. Jack had been sitting where she is before I fell asleep. When I wake up, there she is. I've learned not to question these changings of the guard. I may have been asleep for minutes or days.

Always one to know exactly what to do, Ann begins emptying my vases of stale water and cutting the flowers' stems with the Swiss army knife I always have in my pocketbook. She is bustling about refilling the vases with fresh water and arranging them in the window, leaves and stems all over the floor, when Torch enters my room with the stalk of a general. Jack just told him in the hallway that people from the EP (electrophysiology) lab have been visiting to prepare me for a test.

Torch and Jack don't think I know what they are doing when they disappear into the hall at the same time. I know it means they need to talk privately about me. That's okay. I don't want to know everything. Yet.

Torch is very cross. "You are not undergoing an EP test. We are going to implant a defibrillator without the test. I held your heart in my hands. You could not handle the test. To hell with the insurance companies. They can deal with me."

If he could pound his fist on my soft bed with any result, he would. Ann, covered in petals, looks like she wants to run.

Nice doctors and nurses from the EP lab had been visiting me and giving me brochures to read about how the heart works and why I needed to have some test—a standard procedure, they said, for anyone suspected of having an arrhythmia. I read all their literature about the heart and was grateful to learn more about this organ that I'd taken for granted unless some old boyfriend broke it. I told each conscientious EP visitor that Torch said I did not need the EP test. I thought this was great news because the literature clearly hinted that it was not a pleasant experience.

I didn't realize the bad news: that Torch forbade the test because he was certain that I had recurrent ventricular tachycardia. The EP test could kill me.

Only one to two percent of patients undergoing planned bypass surgery develop ventricular tachycardia, but emergency surgery increases the chances of acquiring this deadly condition. In V-tach, the heart muscle suddenly goes into fibrillation, beating so fast and shallowly that it does not have time to fill up with enough blood for circulation. The result, within a few minutes, is known plainly as sudden cardiac death. This is probably what has occurred when a young athlete dies suddenly during a game or practice.

The good news: I could join the almost 35,000 Americans who had a life-saving defibrillator (also called an implantable cardiac defibrillator or ICD) sewn into the skin above the left breast that year. Leads attached to the heart sense when it is going haywire and send a message to the ICD, which attempts to repace the heart back to a normal rhythm. If the arrhythmia overcomes the repacing function, the defibrillator delivers its "therapy"—a jolt of energy equivalent to about 700 volts (seven times the energy of a 100-watt light bulb). This jolt causes all the muscles in the chest wall to contract and the heart to behave. You may pass out for a minute from the impact, but you're alive.

I am in the EP lab and it is cold and sparkling. I recognize a nurse and two Irish doctors trained at Cork who have been visiting me on Ellison-8. It's a comfort to see a familiar face when you are about to enter the unknown. Lucy makes sure the blankets are nicely tucked in, especially around my toes, which are frigid even in the pink knit slippers they supply. A doctor I do not know, Jeremy Ruskin, director of the cardiac arrhythmia service, comes in. He has kind eyes and talks with me as an equal.

They drape a sheet between my head and my body. This dehumanizes me, making it possible for us to do our jobs, for Jeremy to focus and for me to remain quiet. Nonetheless, I ask questions—using the habit of acquiring knowledge to calm myself, asserting the union of my head behind the sheet with the scrubbed body on the operating table. It's not working. Terror quivers through me. Lucy gives me a Valium and I am weepy. Sloppy, cold tears course out of the corners of my eyes as soft jazz fills the lab like ether. Lucy puts her face close and strokes my forehead.

What the hell am I doing here?

Jeremy administers local anesthesia through a syringe. It pinches and stings deeply. He has to give me several shots because I keep fighting through the anesthesia and feeling the scissors as it cuts the skin above my left breast. Jeremy is creating a pocket between two layers of skin for "the box." It is the size of a small cigarette lighter. I will call it my jewelry box, as it costs $30,000. Thank God for insurance. The box will save my life when I have an arrhythmia, they say. I don't know what they are talking about, though I've read their pamphlets.

On the monitor I watch Jeremy feed the lead from the box through a vein to my heart. I can feel it, just barely. I sense the tugs to my skin as he sews me back up.

So this is what they mean by a noninvasive surgical procedure.

Somehow concentrating through my questions, Jeremy tells me that the battery will run out in about five years, at which point I will undergo another procedure like this one. But research is advancing rapidly, he says. Next time my new device could be the size of a computer chip! I try to express my appreciation when all I feel is horror.

The music switches from melodic jazz to a lovely cello concerto to Celtic ballads. I am crying lightly again from the Valium and from the sadness of it all. Lucy presses close to ask me how I feel.

I feel loved, oddly. She is taking care of me with the close cuddles of a mother next to a crib. She touches a memory.

* * *

The next day, back to the electrophysiology lab I go. It's time to test the box. All my EP friends are here, but I feel like a prisoner-of-war returning to her isolation cell.

They explain the procedure. The test is called NIPS, short for "non-invasive programmed stimulation." It is a dress rehearsal for when ventricular tachycardia hits in real life. After putting me under general anesthesia, first they will mechanically increase my heart rate and see if the box succeeds in repacing the heart back to a normal rhythm. Then to observe the box deliver its "therapy," they will race my heart until it pushes past the repacing function and enters the deadly state of ventricular tachycardia. In case the therapy doesn't work, they have attached the paddles of a big defibrillator to my back, so there is nothing to be afraid of. Nothing at all.

I translate, "So, you'll put me into a death spin and see if the box kicks in, right?"

Right. No one is pleased that I said it like that.

They pour anesthesia into me through my IV and place an oxygen cup over my nose and mouth. I breathe deeply and think nice thoughts as best I can. In a second I am awake again—or so it seems. I resent having to leave the lovely dream, a particularly nice side effect of the anesthesia. They are all happy. The box worked. They did not have to use the big defibrillator; my portable one "delivered its therapy."

So I just died again. Every time this thing goes off, I will die and be resurrected.

Will I ever get used to it? Will it become as natural as sleeping and waking, eating and throwing up? "The box" is now my enemy and my best friend, something it has in common with most essential relationships.

17

I WAKE UP SO SLOWLY. I am a butterfly on the pillow, watching light filter into my room on this quiet morning. At 7 A.M. the phone rings and I struggle to reach for it, careful not to pull off the bandages protecting the incision for the box. Jack calls every morning from his car as he drives to the office, where he'll work until ten. Then he comes to MGH. Mornings are so busy here with eating breakfast, taking pills, and getting washed that visiting any earlier is a waste. I am glad that Tom and the other young doctors are a little late with their rounds today so that the first voice of the day is Jack's.

"I love you, baby," he whispers, and I settle into the pillows for our talk about nothing, feeling like a smitten teenager.

Suddenly, there is a racing jet in my chest. The fast, low rumble. The rapid acceleration. *Oh my God, what is happening?* I look up at my monitor and watch my heart rate shoot in a second from 80 to 260 beats a minute.

BAM.

A horse kicks me in the chest and I drop the phone, shrieking. I hear the rhythmic clanking of plastic on metal. Then pounding. Many feet pounding. The doctors are swarming over me. Wendy is bringing up the rear, running belly forward, yelling "She has a box. She has a box."

Everyone is talking at once. They slap defibrillator pads on me, just in case, and hook me up to an electrocardiogram and begin dialing things. Someone is holding my left hand. It's Stan, Torch's PA minus his Groucho Marx mask. Wendy is on my right. "It's all right, it's all right. Your box worked. You're okay."

"Tell Jack, please someone. He's on the phone." I am breathless, heaving, worrying for Jack. I hear Wendy reassure him and ask him to come. Then she hangs up.

"It's happening again!" I shriek. BAM. I fall back into the pillows, slammed by an invisible assailant—the star of my very own horror movie. I feel only impact, no pain. I have experienced ventricular tachycardia.

They are hooking me up to more IV bags. Joseph, one of the Irish electrophysiologists, appears with a machine and begins swiftly fiddling with it. He explains that he is setting my box to repace irregular heart beats earlier in the game so that I will not need the shock that so violently returns my heart to a normal heart rate. Oh, I get it now. An *implantable* defibrillator.

Jack was on Storrow Drive when he called me. I screamed and he heard the phone clanking against the bed, then many pounding feet, a cacophony of voices. He heard Wendy yelling about the box. He pulled onto a narrow shoulder and stopped, riveted. Cars blasted their horns as they swerved around him. He didn't hear them. He just sat there listening to the radio play starring his wife. Then Wendy spoke to him. He gunned into the traffic, horns blaring, and sped to the hospital. When he walked into my room, he was the picture of calm, making me wonder if I wasn't being a big baby for having hoped he'd come. I was alive, I reasoned, so I must be okay. No big deal.

Then suddenly we were crying and clinging to each other. We had thought I was doing so well. We had thought that the boat was finally leaving this shore of hell.

Marc arrived minutes later. "We tried putting you on a reduced dosage of the drug you've been on to suppress your arrhythmia," he explained. "We've put you back on a higher dosage to give your heart more quiet time to repair itself."

I was all for that. Bring on the drugs! Tylenol with codeine was also recommended to stave off the pain now emanating from the box's pocket in my chest. Take it to stay ahead of the pain, they said.

Jack just left to get some sleep. I am so happy that my sisters Leesa and Becky want to sit and talk with me for a while, even though it is late. Leesa is telling me about the journal she has kept, recording everything as it has happened since May 12: what the doctors said, questions asked and answered, feelings of terror and hope, with dates and times. Others have contributed, too. The result is a mix of hand-writing, a series of misspelled and sometimes mixed-up medical pro-cedures and diagnoses, a painful record of emotional highs and lows.

A brilliant idea. I want to see it. Too soon, too soon, she thinks.

The sound of my nightly dosage of pills rattling in a paper cup announces that Debbie is here. With Debbie and my sisters here, it's a party. She inspires a move to the bathroom, a trained reflex by now when any person in a hospital smock appears.

Stand up slowly. Pause. Try to keep the johnny around my skinny butt as I lean on the IV trolley and we roll across the room. Try to look steadier than I really am in front of my two youngest sisters, who look so helpless in the face of my diminishment. My bowels are churning, pushing. Debbie and I try to pick up the pace. Then she shuts the door and leaves me to work on this privately.

Nothing happens, even though knives are churning in my belly. After fourteen years of doing business in multiple time zones, with morning routines destroyed by airports, car rentals, and meetings at seven, I quickly diagnose the problem.

Goddamned constipation.

I have been such a good girl, drinking prune juice every day, sometimes three times a day. In spite of these prophylactic measures, tonight I am in more pain from this than from any of the other "insults" to my system.

"It's the codeine," Debbie says through the door. "Narcotics can block you up." *Now they tell me.*

"How about an enema?" she offers with alarming enthusiasm.

Oooooooooh, no. I put more spirit into the task at hand. Anything but an enema.

"With everything else you've been through, Deborah, this is nothing. I'm a professional. It doesn't bother me at all. Come on out. We're friends by now; I'm even visiting you in Maine this summer."

That's the point.

Only after a long while do I surrender in desperation. Becky and Leesa politely leave the room on tiptoe, jittery with compassion, shooting me sidelong glances, heads bent as if this will hide my shame. I feel protective. They used to change into their nighties under the bed sheets so I couldn't "see." See what? I'd always wondered.

One hour, one enema, and two suppositories later, and I am still writhing with pain and sweaty cold. My thighs are stuck to the toilet.

"I hate to leave you like this," Debbie coos with eyes like warm blueberries. "My shift is up at eleven and I have a statistics exam tomorrow at eight. There's nothing more that I can do, anyway. It's all a matter of time. Your sisters are here for you."

Are they? Then why did it take a crisis for them to show it, for me to believe it? A banshee shrieks from the depths of my soul and I hush her quickly. *No. Don't go there now—not when there is only love on the other side of the bathroom door.*

Leesa steps up to the door, knocks lightly, and opens it a crack— just enough to be heard, not enough to invade my privacy. She has seen far worse, but I do not understand this yet. Since I lost consciousness, my family has come out from behind the hedges of our youth. I can feel the open space of unconditional love.

"Just rub your stomach, Deb. Rub it and think about the relief you'll feel."

Here I am being coached through the spasms and cold sweats by a sister whose bangs I cut into rick-rack when she was in grammar school. I was always so insistent that I would get it right "this time." And she was always so furious at the pathetic result.

"I'll get you some hot prune juice," Rebecca offers.

I hear my youngest sister pad out of the room decisively to get me exactly what I need in an outside world that I cannot imagine. Becky is larger than life for me in her knowledge of just where to find and warm the prune juice. Is this how she felt long ago when I went into the world beyond our house under the pine trees and returned with red lace-up oxfords for her to wear to first grade? They were just like the ones Mum had bought me ten years before—just like the ones kids with polio wore. She hated them. No polio for her! Becky danced like a fury on the legs now fetching me prune juice.

"Do some visualization. Imagine it all flowing out of you. Let go, let go," Leesa chants without laughing, without embarrassment. I see her squirming under the covers to get her corduroys off and her nightie on. "I swear this works for me, Deborah. I get constipated, too. Keep telling your body to let go."

I think of the snowy image that came to me as I faded away on a gurney at Mount Auburn Hospital. The image was of the only other time in my life I have felt real, life-threatening danger. On a stormy winter day in 1968, when I was sixteen and working after school for Mayo's Pharmacy, I drove down a mountain after delivering medicines to the nursing home. Just as I approached the one-lane bridge across the reservoir, my tires began to skid. Like an automatic emergency announcement, in my mind I heard my father's snow-driving instructions: never brake and resist the skid, but steer into it. I did exactly as he'd taught me. The car fishtailed, then gently sashayed its way to the bridge, straightened out, and sailed gracefully across it. All this took place in winter silence, witnessed only by the falling snow. Hearing Dad's instructions again in my head as I struggled in the emergency room years later may have saved my life; it was an image I took with me as my soul and I retreated deep inside my body to wait out the storm. I'd steered into the skid once again. It dawns on me that both Jack's family and mine have been doing this ever since May 12—letting go of all the brakes on our love.

I close my eyes and let Leesa's soft, low voice carry me away. Becky slips the warm prune juice through the door and I sip slowly as if it were the finest cognac. I put all the old hurt aside, close my eyes, and rub my belly with deep strokes and the concentration of prayer.

"Are you all right?" Leesa cracks the door open farther with "Are you crying?" written on her face.

And finally the exquisite release comes. All those toxins flowing out of my body, out of my soul. The irony is not lost on me and I begin to laugh hysterically.

I emerge from the battle, vainglorious, pale, sheepish. The intimacy makes us a little shy with each other. But we cannot stop the laughter, the giggling relief. Then they tuck me into bed and I want to ask for a story.

We are close again, or maybe for the first time, because now we choose to be. The threat of everlasting separation has united us as it did thirty-two years ago when our mother died. But this time no one is shrugging it off or too young to remember. This time no one can deny its impact on all of us. We are each other's witnesses.

It seemed every time I opened my eyes from a nap, one of my sisters was at my side. We laughed and talked with a freedom I had never experienced with my siblings. At thirteen, fate had given me the unwelcome role of their leader when I hadn't yet gone anywhere myself. They resented me, but I hated myself more. Now, thirty-two years after my mother had died, my recovery seemed to have broken a spell, for my family as well as Jack's.

But this is not a fairy tale. As I recovered, my brother withdrew again—although I had reached into the air from my hospital bed and cupped his cheek, a gesture as universal as waving a white flag. And this is the point: people react to illness and death as they do to their own birthdays—differently and often surprisingly. Confronting mortality takes inner peace, something that was certainly not taught to my generation in grammar school. We practiced piano and baseball, in my case under duress.

One of my oldest, dearest friends said that she didn't "feel much empathy for sick people." I just stared at her, too shocked to react. Revealing the depth of her own vulnerability and denial, her own terror, she went on to say, "Of *course* you're alive—you're young and strong."

There were other astonishments. A woman who had left our friendship in a huff years before sent two loving, supportive notes to my hospital room that arrived when I needed them most. I have no idea how she even knew that I was sick or where I was.

Another friend who writes thank-you notes after the most casual, impromptu clinking of martinis never contacted us at all and seemed to be avoiding us. In fact he later said as much; he just couldn't handle it at the time because of a tragedy in his own family. He was too broken down. And then he felt paralyzingly guilty.

And I understand.

I understand because I have reacted to illness in less-than-perfect ways myself. Abominably, in fact. When my friend Larry was dying of AIDS, I threw a dinner party for him when he was fragile and leaving us, but I never went to see him in his final days. I simply couldn't because I blamed him for his illness, even in the face of his tireless efforts with the AIDS Action Committee in Boston. I was not a good friend. People will give what they can when they can, and it has nothing to do with the love they feel for the patient. It has everything to do with the state of their own souls at the time.

A cold, crinkling sound, like water poured over ice cubes, announces her before I turn my head. The crinkling is from the thin plastic grocery sack she is carrying, wrinkled from being jammed in her kitchen drawer and weighted from something in the bottom of it. Jack has repeatedly asked that no one from work visit me, yet here is the person with whom I worked most closely. I can feel my open heart closing up, the old tension squeezing oxygen that I so desperately need right out of the room. How many years did I work without breathing?

She says with satisfaction that she is glad to see that her flowers on the windowsill are the largest. Her displays of affection have always been a point of confusion for me because I've wanted to believe them. But this time, with the instinct of an animal, I know why she is here and I ask her to go to the locker where my yoga clothes hang and bring me my pocketbook.

Minutes later, when Jack arrives for his morning visit, he sees us with heads bent over our calendars. She protests that this was my idea and that she knows it's not the right time. But I know it is. This moment is the culmination of what our relationship has always really been: a transaction. I have been useful, and now I am not.

Reviewing my calendar, I empty my life of any future commitments to meetings and strategic plans, flight numbers and departure times, sales presentations and conference calls. I've met my last deadline and it's over. Reciting names and dates from the calendar, my recall of the details connected to pencil scratchings next to every hour of every day for months on end is extraordinary. Jack tries to stop me as I hammer all the information I have out of my brain. But no one can stop me now. My former life is flying off the pages.

When I am done, Jack announces that I am tired and the visit is over. She leaves me the grocery bag. Inside is an orange.

After Jack has walked her to the door he comes back to my side and finds me panting, eyes wild. He holds my hand and says, "You will never work again, Deborah, I promise. Never again."

But I know he is really telling me that I *can* never work again. My heart cannot handle it.

18

CALLIE IS BRINGING my eleven-year-old nephew Chris to visit this afternoon! Callie was about Chris's age when she last saw our mother in the hospital, so I want to be sure I look good for her son because I am going to live. I remember how critically I perused Mother's wasted body, missing nothing, especially not the smells. I get out of bed all by myself and roll the IV trolley to the bathroom without buzzing anyone for help, toting a bag of toiletries.

After wandering into the room a few times without seeing me, Wendy notices that I have been in the bathroom for longer than normal. She calls to me through the door but doesn't hear my answer, so she cracks it open.

I turn to her, my face green as a reptile, and she screams, then collapses back on my bed clutching her big belly, howling.

Once my facial is rinsed off and my skin is glowing, Wendy brings me some makeup. I put blusher on my cheeks and check every angle of my face for anything that would scare Chris. Then I try to comb the tangle of wild hair billowing around my face, finally managing to hoist it up with a few clips into something resembling my Katharine Hepburn look. Wendy fixes one of the clips because it is shooting a clump of hair straight up like a feather headdress. Do I want to shuffle back into the bathroom to get a better look? Too tired. It won't matter. Chris always thinks my hair is messy anyway. I put on perfume and hitch the johnny up to my throat, cupping the excess underarm fabric in my armpit to hold the front more modestly across my chest. In time Chris will see the scar, just not now.

He approaches my bed shyly in his after-school soccer uniform, proud to be on the team and wanting the whole hospital to see. I smile like the old days, but the flash isn't there and he knows it. You can't fool a sensitive kid. All by himself at the Ipswich five-and-dime, he bought me a small teddy bear for company. He places it now on my table. After some initial awkwardness, my skinny favorite boy climbs into bed with me, trying out the automatic buttons and riding the ocean swells with me, laughing and clowning like before. For a few minutes,

normal everyday life peeks into my room and I have the freshly mois-
turized face to prove it.

It was around this time, in private hallway conversations with Torch
and Marc, that Jack began to lobby for my convalescence in Maine
after a month's transition in Boston, during which time we would live
with our friends Juliana and Mark, three blocks from the hospital.
My doctors argued against a move to Maine this soon. They said that
more arrhythmias were very likely in my future, so I should stay in
Boston. Jack argued that our own apartment would be too isolating.
In Maine the water, weather, and mountains would be at my door; I
would be part of life, not cut off from it. Jack believed in the medicine
of smelling my garden and watching it wake up. Besides, we have a
small hospital in our town with a helicopter pad, making it possible to
get to Mass General faster than I'd get there in rush-hour traffic. And
Maine would attract a constant flow of "babysitters"—friends from
"away" (Maine's term for anyone who does not go back generations
in town) who would look after me while Jack was working in Boston. Jack also argued that my long-term care would be easier in Maine
because neighbors would be able to keep a constant, gentle lookout for
me without disrupting their lives.

Jack is willful when he gets an idea into his head, especially if I
agree. At first, the doctors did not like our proposal at all; I was still
in my acute phase, each day an uncharted sea. They wanted only my
recovery and safety. They wanted to be sure that I would live and
maybe even thrive.

So did Jack.

As usual, one morning Jack's assistant, Judy, rode the elevator to the
third floor of Genzyme. She liked being the first one in the department. But these days she barely got any work done; she was always
fielding phone calls about me and worrying about Jack. Without Judy,
Jack wouldn't have eaten even the half-a-sandwich that sustained him
each day.

She put down her bag and started her computer, scanning the
day's schedule. Then she realized that there were voices coming from

Jack's office. The door was slightly ajar and she knocked lightly as she opened it a little wider to see who was there.

A gray rubber body was on the floor and Jack was straddling it, jacket off, tie askew. A young woman was telling Jack to place his mouth on the dummy's and breathe while rhythmically pumping the dummy's chest.

Judy's first instinct was to giggle. Then she backed out in tears. She had forgotten that today was Jack's CPR training.

Jack planned for my discharge with the same meticulousness he brought to his expeditions. All his life he's had what he calls his "airplane dreams"—nightmares, actually—of a plane crash when he is frantically saving everyone. He is the hero, the only one who can do it. Now Jack was living the nightmare he'd prepared for: our plane had crashed and he was doing everything he could to keep me alive.

The Big Guy, or TBG, helped Jack in setting up a safety network. That's Dave, the six-foot-six head of Genzyme security and a former cop, nicknamed by Jack. TBG had begun by finding a CPR instructor to come to Jack's office and give him a three-hour refresher course. To persuade the doctors to approve my move to Maine, TBG had one of his men drive from Boston to our door, mapping the routes to every hospital along the way and compiling a book of exits and directions to keep in our car. Then he found a beeper system for Jack to wear whenever he left me so that we could be in constant contact in case I chose that moment to die on him. One system was so high-tech that it connected us to Moscow, but it was useless in our small town. They opted for two systems: one beeper for when Jack was outside Maine, another for when he drove into town for milk.

They are moving me from my bed onto a gurney for a ride through the hospital, lifting me over the' crevasse that drops far below to the linoleum floor. I ride through the wide, wide hospital world until we enter a lab where a pleasant young man in green rolls me under a machine that looks like a torpedo.

I am in the nuclear medicine lab and my ejection fraction (EF) is to be tested, now that it has had almost three weeks to rise. The EF is a vital measure of the heart's strength, based on the rate at which it pumps blood through its chambers. I look into my body and will it to do well. After all, I am walking without leaning on the IV trolley for five minutes three times a day every day. I can also talk, eat, read, and laugh. These are, I think, all signs of great improvement.

The young man in green is not succeeding in taking a blood sample. I have learned that I am a "hard stick": my blood has been taken so many times that my veins have become thick as leather.

"I think I'd better see if someone else can help us," he says with sweaty relief. I relax a bit.

A pro enters and swiftly takes a blood sample for a benchmark. Then he injects me with a small amount of radioactive fluid, and I lie there while it enters my bloodstream. When it is well mixed with my own blood, they take multiple pictures from three directions at three ten-minute intervals. I must lie still, still, still—I make sure I scratch my nose before we begin. Then I look up at the ceiling and go far away. I fly through that ceiling to lie in my hammock with the breeze rocking the huckleberry bushes and me. Then I push off from a frozen shore and skate down the lake at a furious speed.

What am I doing lying under a torpedo as if my life depends on it?

The next morning I am desperate, hungry for Jack.

"Oh please, please, please! It's okay. There's plenty of room. Look, I can squish over here and you can come in."

I squiggle to one side of the bed, pushing IV trolleys out of the way. It's been weeks since I have felt my husband's body next to mine, and I cannot stand it another minute.

Jack is shy with me. He takes off his blazer. "You're sure? I won't hurt you?"

He lowers the metal handles on one side of the bed and gets in gingerly, as though he is lying in broken glass. He keeps his shoes on in case he needs to make a quick getaway.

Oh *happiness*.

Just feeling the warmth of his skin through his shirt fills me with strength. We giggle like kids doing something wonderfully naughty. Jack relaxes his body, sort of; I can feel the muscles in his arms go slack, though he's still holding his chin like a marine at attention. I close my eyes and inhale his scent.

"Would you like me to come back later?" Marc Semigran is half-way into the room and clearly embarrassed.

Giddy with joy, I am reckless for a minute and say, "No, please come in, Marc. We just finished, so you're not interrupting anything."

Jack shoots me one of his looks, gets up, and shakes Marc's hand solemnly. They sit by my bed.

Marc's cheeks are still a little pink. He is struggling to say something. We wait as he delivers a careful introduction. And then he says it.

"I got your results from the nuclear medicine lab. Your ejection fraction has not budged much. It is at 25 percent and unlikely to move any higher. The greatest gains are in the first three weeks following surgery. There may be some more movement in the next few months, but we can't count on that."

He cannot hide his disappointment. I know he was as buoyed as we were by my apparent progress.

I look from Marc to Jack, but I feel vacant. *So, I have half a heart to work with. Even couch potatoes have EFs of at least 50 percent.*

Jack becomes an old man before my eyes, like one of those speeded-up nature films that depict the entire life of a caterpillar in a couple of seconds.

"You have cardiomyopathy, Deborah," Marc says with resignation. "A large part of your left ventricle is dead, the muscle tissue severely damaged. There is no getting it back."

I am not surrendering. "But why am I doing so well?"

"The rest of your body is in good shape and it's bearing the brunt. You came here an otherwise very healthy woman from a lifetime of good habits."

"I think of all the potato chips I could have eaten . . . I guess it wouldn't have made a difference."

"Oh, it would have made a difference," Marc says pointedly. "You would be dead."

And if I were dead, I would not be *here* on this hospital bed, having just felt the warmth of my husband's body. I shift from disappointment to gratitude, quickly.

19

"TODAY YOU'RE GOING TO LEARN ABOUT YOUR DRUGS."

Wendy is sitting on my bed, her pregnant belly draped so far over the edge that I fear she will tumble to the floor like Humpty Dumpty. I haven't quite thought of my tiny colored pills as drugs. They seem so benign. I can't imagine learning about them—there are too many. And besides, why bother? I trust the nurses.

"It's not an issue of trust. You need to know what you are ingesting when you go home."

Go home? I can't possibly go home yet. And then it hits me.

"You mean I have to keep taking these drugs?"

"Yes, Deborah." Wendy looks a little surprised at my question, then realizes that I am adrift in confusion.

"For how long?"

"Probably for a long time." She holds my hand and I search her eyes.

"How long is a long time?"

"Like most of your life." She looks me square in the eye.

I am still again. *So this is not going away.* I take as many pills in a single day as I used to take vitamins in a week. Another change, another milestone.

She goes through the list: potassium, Lasix, baby aspirin, digoxin, Coumadin, Vasotec, and amiodarone. Tylenol with codeine in case I need it for pain. It will be overwhelming to keep track of the side effects from these drugs: constipation, hair loss, bruising, bleeding in the lungs and stomach, hemorrhages, the leaching of essential potassium, diarrhea, blurred vision, loss of appetite and interest in sex, dizziness, lightheadedness, sensitivity to sunlight, itching, stomach upset, ringing in the ears, rapid heart rate, slow pulse rate, skin rash, breast enlargement. She pauses when she gets to amiodarone.

"This is a very strong drug, a heart suppressant, that you really need now. But it's a bummer. People should not be on it more than six months to a year, or you run the risk of damage to other organs, like the lungs, liver, and thyroid. It can cause lung scarring, for example. Watch your skin carefully for a bluish tint."

I am not absorbing this. I am pulling down a veil through which I can peek at her. How could they possibly give me a drug that hurts me?

"Why do I need this drug, Wendy?"

"You have ventricular tachycardia. That's what caused your box to go off the other day. You've sustained numerous insults to the heart and it's irritated. The electrical system is shot . . ."

She's lost me already.

She sighs. "OK. Let's pretend you, in your car, are an electrical impulse and your heart's chambers are the highway. To drive to Maine, you have to go through several tollbooths." She shifts her body and warms to the analogy. "Now, on the other side of each tollbooth the road is all torn up and bumpy. That's the damage to your heart muscle. If your car hits those bumps, it will jumble around and crash, maybe killing you, right? So amiodarone is like dark glasses. If you wear sunglasses, you can't see the bumps, and your electrical impulses sail right through to the next toll booth." She looks at me triumphantly, hopefully.

I think it's brilliant. Sunglasses for the heart. Just what I need.

"Ready to get rid of those staples?"

Dr. George Tolis strolls in with a simple pair of tweezers. He is the resident who has most often been assigned to me. On his days off he comes to the hospital to do paperwork dressed in soft flannel shirts and wide-wale corduroys. He visits me then, too, and I see a hint of the Greek sun that would shine in his classic face if he weren't so tired.

I am thrilled to be rid of the staples but horrified at the prospect of having them pulled out. George moves swiftly, starting at my crotch. I am deeply embarrassed and repulsed. This last vestige of modesty surprises me. I close my eyes until he's done a few, then watch. The nerve endings have not reconnected through my scar yet, so I am happily numb. I feel only little tugs as each staple is neatly lifted and discarded.

George chats nicely as though it is the most normal thing in the world for a woman to spread her legs so that he can attack her with tweezers. Then it's over and he has preserved my dignity somehow. I learn that he was in the operating room with me and that he was the hero who removed the endotracheal tube from my throat. Now he has rescued me from the staples. Their imprint on my red scar makes my leg look like a grotesque version of George's wide-wale corduroy pants.

"Want to go home today?" Marc smiled broadly as he entered the room while I contentedly ate breakfast, watching light dance and the world go by on the Charles River.

I was stunned, panicked. No, I don't want to go home. How can I live without any of you?

Marc gave me one more day in the hospital, enough time for us to put together a plan. It would begin with a move down the street to Juliana's and Mark's apartment on Beacon Hill. Callie took charge of organizing round-the-clock care for the next few weeks by friends and family, in addition to visiting nurses.

On June 4, Jack and Wendy helped me give away my flowers. Plants to the man who delivered my supper and loved to garden. Flower bouquets for the main desk and for Wendy to take home. A special one set aside for Debbie, whose shift began later. My sneakers to Michelle, my favorite technical aide in the SICU—a perfect fit for a larger-than-life woman. I began crying when Miss Aida came to say goodbye. She was the beloved mother of the floor who had delivered lunch every day with the rolling grace of a grand ship. She called everyone darling, but I took her affectionate words as if they were for me alone, the perfect antidote to technology and terror.

Torch was finally off on the vacation he had postponed for months, so Marc officiated at my discharge. He responded thoroughly and with mild amusement to what had become my daily question-and-answer session, each one dated and numbered in my notebook along pale gray lines that gave order to internal chaos. My parting notes looked something like this:

- *Chance of another heart attack?* Highly unlikely given that the damage is in the area affected by the artery only. Overall immediate health will depend on the ventricular function.

- *Baths?* Wait until after the ICD bandage is removed and Jeremy says OK.

- *Incisions?* All healing nicely. Don't get sun on scars or they will deepen. Scabs mean they are still not healed so NO CREAM until Torch says OK.

- *Needlelike pain in heart area?* Just fine, means healing.

- *Food?* Low-fat, low-salt, low-cholesterol. Ethnic food in moderation. NO green tea of any kind including peppermint. Eat consistent amounts of vitamin K foods—leafy greens are natural blood thickeners that counteract Coumadin, an anticoagulant.

- *Self-monitor?* Watch for fluid retention, fatigue, and breathlessness. Weigh myself every day. A gain of just two pounds in two days or swelling in the hands or feet means the meds are not working. Wake up, pee, weigh. Watch bumps and bruises—can easily lead to hemorrhaging.

- *Activity?* Can go up and down stairs, but rest if dizzy or lightheaded. Only restricted by what I can't tolerate. No extreme moves on left arm so the ICD lead does not pull out of heart. But don't keep it so still that shoulder locks.

- *Driving?* No driving for at least six months because we don't know yet if arrhythmia is stable. If box went off, could endanger self and others.

- *Medications?* For pain or colds, regular Tylenol is OK. TAKE NOTHING WITHOUT ASKING. Do not skip heart medications. Miss one, just go on to the next—don't double-medicate. Call.

- *Reminders about the box:* Keep distance from cell phones, radio antennas, some automatic garage doors, heavy machinery, power lines, airport security scanners, and anything with an electromagnetic field. (Does a flashlight have an electromagnetic field? Ask Jack.)

- *Reminders:* Certainly no running, no climbing stairs swiftly, no swimming, no skiing, no skating, no bicycling. Do not pull, push, shove, lift. Never shovel or vacuum. No hanging out the laundry. Walk and rest every day.

- *No, no, no, no . . .*

"Above all, never ignore how you feel," Marc told me. "Report any aches and pains, and be sure to tell me if the box goes off."

I felt like a student cramming for an exam who barely grasped any of the material.

"Tell me again, Marc. Tell me exactly what is wrong with me," I said.

He patiently repeated that I had two serious heart conditions: cardiomyopathy and ventricular tachycardia, damaged muscle tissue and a deadly heartbeat. I scribbled the words in my notebook and stared at them for a while.

"But you're alive, Deb," he said, reminding me of the important thing.

Terror is shivers in a hot room and frozen glances and pretense. I hoped a brave smile would mask it.

Time to go. I stand by my bed in familiar old clothes that feel strange. Jack brought sweatpants, my beat-up running shoes, and a soft, long-sleeved cotton T-shirt that would not chafe my tender skin. I throw my arms around Marc and cling for dear life. He tolerates my embrace with confusion and embarrassment. Doesn't know where to put his hands. Wants this display to be over fast.

I can't think of any way to thank him adequately for giving the world back to me. I believe that I will never see him again. I still don't understand that we are wedded forever, and so I give him the best gift

I can think of: a wish for great love at home for his whole life. It feels Chinese, ancient, ultimate. Marc looks at me, puzzled, then his eyes turn to curved slits, reminding me of my first sense of him from my bed in the SICU, when I thought he was a cartoon.

Jack tucks me into a wheelchair and pushes me into the corridor. I am a bag of bones embarking on high adventure. The main station on Ellison-8 is a blurry mass of people waving goodbye. Wendy's belly is all that is distinct in the mist.

As the big aluminum elevator doors close with a dull whump, separating me from Ellison-8, I tremble at the thought of returning to life without the people of MGH. My ICD is a souvenir, like rosary beads from Italy in a tiny mosaic box. We wheel slowly through the hospital past areas that I have not been able to imagine. Gift shops, newsstands, coffee shops, pharmacies, rest rooms, information booths. It is a whole city. People bustle—no, they run. People stare. I smile triumphantly.

We push through the main doors and I hold my breath through curling cigarette smoke from patients inhaling in desperate, short gasps while leaning on IV trolleys. Beyond their haze is a merry-go-round of taxis and whistles. Summer has begun and my first breath of fresh air in a month brings rain and sun deep into my lungs. I *am alive*.

SUMMER

20

BOSTON SKIPPED RIGHT OVER SPRING THAT YEAR, as I had. June's temperatures soared abruptly from damp cold to searing heat. In my protected, air-conditioned cage above Beacon Hill, I learned how to do normal things again, very slowly, mindful of the energy it took simply to be. Each day was filled with small triumphs. I learned to grip my toothbrush and to step over the edge of the bathtub, with Jack holding me as though we were dancing the polka. Eventually I had my first shower without Jack's assistance, holding on to the towel rack for dear life.

In a week I could stand up in the shower and close my eyes without toppling over while the water ran all over my numb back and I shielded the bandages for the ICD above my left breast. One day Jack caught me balancing on one foot while I carefully washed the other. He stared, afraid to move. I was the great blue heron who visits our cove every summer—poised on a spindly leg, staring fixedly at the water for fish, ready to fly away at the blink of an eyelash.

I stayed on the main floor all day, enjoying the company of babysitters while resting on the couch and watching the color of the apartment walls change as the sun made its way across Boston's skyline. I walked in circles through the apartment for five, then ten minutes, three times a day—my graduation assignment from physical therapy. I would finish two minutes and ask Jack if I was done yet. He hid his despair and coached me patiently.

I could not open a door by myself. The exertion was simply too much for my lungs and chest. To increase the capacity of my lungs, I blew and blew into the lung toy the nurses had given me, trying to get the capsule to rise to the top. It seemed impossible.

When I was alone, I talked with Gracie, Juliana's parrot, to whom I was allergic. As I lurched and sneezed my way around the apartment, Gracie yoo-hooed and sang the first few bars of "Misty." She became very cranky and loud if I ignored her, especially at nap times. She made me laugh. And gag. Gracie's beautiful cage was filled with tidbits of food and brightly colored toys—rings and ladders to climb on, perches from which she could observe the world and chatter. When Juliana came home from work, she would place Gracie on her shoulder and give her a ride wherever she went in the apartment. Outside of her cage, Gracie eyed me with suspicion. I didn't blame her. Being on the outside was scary.

Juliana bought me a flat plastic box with twenty-eight compartments labeled "SUN MON TUE WED THU FRI SAT" across the top and "MORN NOON EVE BED" down the side. Into these compartments we organized my medication for each week, nine pills a day. The level of detail was overwhelming; the pills were pink, white, apricot, and yellow, round, square, oval, and hexagonal. We had to squint to see the differences. Using our fingernails, we split some of the pills in half to get the right dosage, following the instructions in my discharge booklet. I sleepwalked through the whole sorting exercise, fighting to concentrate. My struggle was emotional; I simply could not believe that I had to live every day with this many drugs. My jaw clenched in resentment every time I snapped open one of the box's little compartments and shook the pills into my hand. I never took the Tylenol with codeine the hospital had given me for pain; it was far more painful to accept the drugs that were now my life's companions. I could not tolerate the idea of even one more pill. Or of another bout with constipation.

For a change of pace, my sister Callie drove me to a drugstore to buy a pill-splitter. Beside us, an elderly lady was comparing various kinds and trying to decide which one was right for her. She looked up at me, dressed in my baggy dress, and said, "Oh, congratulations! I remember the pills they gave me when I was your age and pregnant, too. Wait until you grow old and see how many you have to take then!"

I was speechless at her joyful assumption—at the fraud of my youth, at my body's betrayal. I thanked her and we fled as fast as I could wobble.

Like the June flowers that have not quite declared themselves as they emerge from their ground cover, my appetites began to poke through haltingly, beginning with food. During my hospital stay, our friend Hillery had tried to coax my taste buds to life by bringing me a thermos of real chicken soup, a colorful ceramic Italian bowl, and a silver soupspoon. I could barely taste her perfect offering, but I knew it was good from the velvety texture and from memories of eating well at her table. My tongue was still too bruised from the intubation process to enjoy flavor. It was also bumblingly useless while I ate messy foods like a tuna sandwich—it couldn't sweep my teeth clean, a reflex I appreciated for the first time. I tried not to smile after lunch until I had brushed my teeth. It was on Beacon Hill that I ate my first real meals, small portions of dishes that the others tore into. I even had a thimble of red wine once. It did not taste good, but I vaguely remembered enjoying it before.

In time, I was able to walk up and down the stairs of the apartment slowly. I added this to my training program, motivated by the physical therapist's prescription for sex: two flights of stairs with no breathlessness. Though my sexual appetite had fled along with my huge appetite for food, I wanted to be prepared just in case.

One boiling day, when I knew everyone would return from work drenched in sweat, I found leeks, potatoes, and low-fat milk in the refrigerator and decided to make vichyssoise for a cool supper. Noting with satisfaction that I had advanced from holding a pencil to holding a knife, I chopped happily, if awkwardly. A task that once would have taken me half an hour took almost all morning, but it was worth it—a delicious harbinger of a life with chores and pleasures in the kitchen. When Juliana saw my masterpiece chilling in the refrigerator, she expressed amazement, then admonished me for overexerting myself. The act of cooking was monumental, but at the time it did not feel that way to me. It was an old reflex that I had rediscovered, like standing on one foot.

That night at the dinner table, Juliana dissolved into tears while looking straight at me as though I had punched her.

"I just couldn't imagine life without you."

Always protective of others, Juliana hides her sorrows behind the smile of your very bestest friend in kindergarten. In seventeen years of friendship I had never seen her cry, and now she was bawling. *She would miss me if I were dead.* This hadn't occurred to me. When you are sick, your world is in such disarray that you re-create it as a bee builds a hive, cell by cell from the inside out. Eventually you make it from the interior of your body to your mind, at which point you might begin to grasp the suffering of others.

The truth is that it is far more difficult emotionally to observe someone who is sick and dying than it is to be the patient. Friends and family are the people who actually experience the death, not those who die. The helplessness of those who would do anything but cannot is torturous. My body was the center of an explosion to which I had no choice but to surrender. Family and friends were left violently reeling, too, but they never got to wear the hospital gown that signals "Be gentle with me because I am in trouble." After the crisis, they were expected to reenter the world as though nothing had happened, unscathed. But that was a lie.

My sister Becky was the first to return to work. She drove back to Connecticut a couple of days after I regained consciousness and commuted to Boston on weekends. She remembers looking through the windshield as she drove out of Boston and seeing cumulus clouds against a brilliant blue sky. She wept at their beauty, a miracle that would have been only a detail on the Mass Pike in the days before time stopped for all of us. On her first day in the office, no one spoke to her about what she'd just been through. No one asked how I was, or whether I had lived or died. Her colleagues intended no harm; no one knew what to say besides, "Hi, Becky. Coffee's on." She went back to designing in a daze, staring at mockups uncomprehendingly. *Does it really matter if that line is straight? If it's blue or red?* The project in front of her—designing Christmas packaging for a new beer—seemed surreal.

Becky was not the only one who had trouble returning to the outside world. It was difficult for everyone who had been with me at the epicenter. In the hospital every moment had been charged with vitality. Vitality—the expression of life force—is perhaps an odd word to use in connection with illness. Yet even when I was near death, there had been a holiday atmosphere around my bed. People let go of everyday concerns, which they knew in their hearts did not really matter. Once the desperate vigil was over, it was hard to break the spell and live life in an ordinary way again, to squander seconds.

Many people, from intimates to total strangers who heard the story third-hand, took my illness like a bonk over the head and reassessed their lives. There were marriages and divorces. People retired, changed jobs, switched careers, moved. Our friend Steven was the quickest off the block. He quit his job in New York; laid the groundwork to move back to Boston, closer to many of his dearest friends; then traveled to Turkey, a country he'd always wanted to see. My sister Leesa resigned from a job that involved endless turmoil, took a few months off to repair her body and soul, and found a new job with what she really valued: *nice people*. Becky entered a period of deep reflection on personal and artistic fulfillment and put a plan in motion for change. Even Callie, whose demanding life left little time for personal reflection and fun, found herself thinking about taking painting classes and visiting the Museum of Fine Arts more than once a year. Just thinking about it was monumental.

Sometimes the reassessments were involuntary. One day, Ann was paged during a meeting. The hapless caller reported that a marketing campaign would be held up by a week. Ann, beloved by her colleagues for her even temper and her kindness, became enraged.

"Don't ever call me with news like this as though it is an emergency," she yelled into the phone. "It is not an emergency. Do you understand? This is not an emergency. They are shoes. Only shoes."

Seven pairs of eyes around a polished conference table stared at her. The incident triggered a good, hard look at how soulless she'd been feeling in her job, and she began to think about starting her own business so *she* could decide what mattered. It opened in February 2001.

Jack returned to work for half-days and the routine was good for him. Wherever he went, people came out of their offices to greet him. He had the physical sensation of being carried by them as they walked down hallways at his side, asking after me, asking about him. His epiphany was to believe in their love, which he had dared to make a priority for Genzyme's culture when he became the first human resources officer. People were not afraid to show affection, to cry. But Jack couldn't always see the faces he smiled at so nicely, because at any moment he might get The Call. All phones were ringing for him. He became a nervous fist, clenching and releasing.

My epiphany happened in an unlikely place. One Saturday, Jack took me to a day spa for a haircut, followed by a pedicure, an indulgence I had never experienced. It was Callie's idea, of course. She said that red polish on my toes was just the medicine I needed. A massage was out—my foot was the only part of my body on which I was allowed to put oil. One by one I climbed the stairs to the second floor, eschewing the elevator in a fit of determination. I held fast to the railing and walked up two or three stairs, then rested. Jack looked deep into my face to read the inside of my body. When I was ready, I attempted the next three stairs. And so we made it to the top, only five minutes late for my appointment. The whole staff was standing in the window applauding. I felt like Sylvester Stallone in the movie *Rocky* and shot a bony fist into the air, grinning. The staff made a nice fuss over me and had clearly told the other patrons about my illness because they joined in the cheer, too.

Except for one woman. She kept her back to me as I made my way into the room and slipped out of the manicure section as I was being seated in the chair to have my hair washed. I saw her in the mirror, though, and she did not speak to me, though our eyes locked for a second with recognition. She was a woman I knew through work. We'd had lunch twice. She was always impeccably dressed, and now I knew why her hands were intimidatingly flawless, making me hide my scruffy nails cut blunt and short, ready for the next plunge into dishwater or garden soil. Her swift slap of indifference stung. I was no longer useful to her. She paid quickly and fled.

Or had she simply not recognized me in my state of pure spirit, stripped of my skill at being in the world, incapable of trying to please people like her anymore? Or better, not caring to?

One positive side effect of being sick is a swift sorting of priorities. Illness, oddly enough, can give life back to us.

21

THE ELEVATOR OPENS and Callie steps into Juliana's and Mark's apartment, cheery and organized, masking her tension well. We are going back to the hospital for my first visit as an outpatient—first to the anticoagulation unit for training in monitoring Coumadin, a blood thinner, and then to the EP lab for a checkup of my jewelry box.

Even though Marc Semigran has sternly told me that my chest cannot handle carrying, pushing, or pulling anything for months—and I know this because I am too weak anyway—we have to negotiate the process of getting me out of the apartment, into the elevator, through two heavy doors, and out to the stoop to wait for the cab, avoiding the sun because of my skin's new drug-induced photosensitivity. As Callie predicted, it is difficult for me, the bossy older sister, to refrain from pathetic attempts to help her orchestrate our passage downstairs. She leaves me on the stoop for a moment while she resets the burglar alarm, and I am in trouble already. A carpenter who is working on the building looks so hot and tired, I offer to refill his water bottle. As I say the words, I know I am insane. Callie gives me a look as she takes his bottle and goes back upstairs. I am ready for my scolding in the cab.

"You may never, never do that again. This is all about *you* now, Deborah. Other people's needs don't matter. How stupid could he be to come to a job site on a scorching day with only one water bottle? That is his problem, not yours. Besides, you don't even know that guy. By what little you said, he now knows that you are sick and weak and often alone upstairs."

She is steamier than the day. She is also right. The realization is more jarring and uncomfortable than the lurching, lumpy backseat of the cab. *So, I have to rethink everything, then, don't I?* I no longer have energy to squander, so I can take no impulse for granted. I have to reconstruct my approach to the world, just as Callie and I mapped out a whole strategy for simply getting to the door.

I think of my move to Switzerland in 1974 to teach at an international boarding school in a tiny village where women had just gotten voting rights. How did I adjust? I watched as much as I could until I learned the language and the rules. My first lesson came on a street corner in Lucerne when the firm hand of an old lady pulled me back by the belt of my dress. In Switzerland, pedestrians are forbidden to cross the street against the signal, even with no traffic in either direction for several blocks, even if you have just arrived from America with a pack on your back and confusion in your eyes.

I am newly arrived in the land of the sick. I am simply learning the rules.

Callie helps me out of the cab in front of the hospital and we walk a few feet before I am dizzy from all the commotion. It is too soon to show off my walking skills, too soon to stride in with triumph that I do not yet feel and cannot fake. I grab on to a post, the rapids rushing around me. At last she finds me a wheelchair and I collapse into the brown vinyl seat. Much better. Too much excitement already. We wheel into the hospital and I want to move back in. Life was safe here.

Callie is doing a masterful job with the wheelchair, until we have to turn a corner. Then the wheels spin and stick, and we giggle. I love being with her, love being protected by the younger sister who has always played out her second-born's role of defiant scamp to my role of fearless (but totally unqualified) leader. It's lovely, this truce, for both of us, I think, I hope. But Callie rarely shares her feelings, so I'll never know.

Suzanne is my anti-coagulation unit caseworker and introduces herself with warm efficiency. This is the lab to which my weekly blood samples will be sent for testing.

Weekly blood samples?

On reflection I realize that someone has probably said this to me before, like everything else. I sneak a look at my bruised and dotted hands and arms. They look like a junkie's.

I hate having my blood drawn, having any needle even within eyesight. I remember the IV ladies with their clinking trays arriving in the wee hours of the morning, summoned by desperate technical aides when my needle needed changing. The IV ladies were an odd pair, like Cockney walk-ons in My Fair Lady, one large and plain, one small and painted brilliantly. They spoke in close succession, as though they were one person.

"Now just hold still while I take this old one out."

"Oh, yes, dearie me. You are swollen."

"Good thing you spoke up."

"Oh, dear, however will we get a new one in?"

"Don't you worry, dear."

"You slap, slap, slap the arm, you see, dear."

"The younger girls are afraid to do this and hurt the patients, aren't they?"

"Yes they are. But multiple sticks hurt more, don't they?"

"Ah, yes they do."

And I'd be swiftly retaped to the needles in my arms before they rattled off, talking over each other in indistinguishable murmurs.

Suzanne launches into all the dos and don'ts of my new life on Coumadin. I take notes furiously. She hands me a pamphlet. The meeting is over—she thinks.

"Suzanne, may I review with you all the immediate actions you've just given me?"

I read back to her the ten key items that I need to do right away, which I have distilled from the mass of details. She gives me an astonished "A." I marvel that they repeat this list for each new patient. Then she tells me that they are monitoring three thousand patients a year with a skeletal staff. Summoning up the old management-consultant Deborah, I volunteer to send her a copy of the checklist I just wrote. Callie rolls her eyes.

Off to the EP lab we go. In the waiting room we read soft, wrinkled magazines with cover lines like, "You too Can Try a New Look. Here's How." I think about how articles like this fuel women's insecurities and remember feeling ugly at fourteen if I had not applied eyeshadow. Then I copy out a recipe for a dip with nonfat yogurt, cilantro, roasted red peppers, and sun-dried tomatoes. Callie smiles; it's a good sign that food is beginning to get my attention.

Mary, who runs the ICD outpatient program, calls me in. She has bouncy soft brown hair to her shoulders and relaxes me with the right mix of soothing nonchalance and clear explanation. I can tell she does this often. She hooks me up to the ICD testing machine and I hold a paddle over my left breast. Suddenly I feel cold and clammy with misgiving. Callie feels my mood shift from across the room before I do.

Mary explains that she is first going to "interrogate" the box—to read the information stored in my ICD to see if I have had any arrhythmias. Yes, it sure does feel like a nasty interrogation sitting in this hospital chair with wires pasted all over me. She says I will feel nothing, and to hold the paddle steady. Paper rolls out of the machine with tiny printed data, like squished ants. I feel nothing but imagine everything. *Are you finding problems? How bad is it? Is the box working right? What if it's not?* I lock eyes with Callie.

"You're all set!" Mary says cheerfully. "No arrhythmias."

I am alive once more! I soar and feel the wind drying my clammy skin. *So, I can go now.*

"Next we need to increase your heart rate a little to see how the machine reacts."

Sisyphus in Hades, I pick up my rock again with the knowledge that it is never over, never completely good news. Mary has to use a little effort to reposition my hand with the paddle over my heart—sort of like when Barbara Spivak, my general practitioner, gently pries my legs apart for my annual gynecology exam. I try to cooperate and relax.

She fiddles with dials and I feel my heart begin to race in its garage. It rumbles up and lodges in my thorax. It makes me nauseated.

"All right, Deb? This will be over in a minute." She keeps her eyes on the dials.

The controlled, slight rattle that rises to the base of my throat brings back all the memories, the recognition of death, the desperation, the helplessness. It is epic, and over in a minute.

"All set again! Your box works fine."

"How often will we do this, Mary?" I ask, using questions to calm myself.

"Oh, about every three months." *Every three months?*

"For how long?"

"For as long as you have the box in. We have to be sure it is working for you."

Her eyes tell me that she knows this is hard for me to hear, that she is experienced in telling patients that they are tethered for life. I knew that once a year I would return to the EP lab to have my box fully tested, but I had not realized there would be four other scheduled meetings with death annually.

Callie and I are silent as we wheel out. She knows not to show any pity. I'd spit on her if she did. I just need time. *Give me time.*

The cabdriver for the short trip home is surly. I feel my temper rising. He is wasting a day. He has no idea how precious it is to him—let alone to me. Simply because I am in a cab it is an outing, and he is raining on it. When Callie gets out to open the door for me, I lean over the front seat and dump my anger at the gods all over this stranger I will never see again.

"I am dying and you just hurt fifteen minutes of my last days. Do you understand how much a simple, polite hello and goodbye mean?"

He looks startled. Suddenly his English is good. He apologizes sincerely and his whole demeanor shifts to gentleness. Then I am ashamed. Maybe he has learned to put on an indifferent, tough face to do his job. Maybe he is suffering and just can't be cheerful anymore. My little fit tells me that I have not yet absorbed my first lesson: leave the world behind—just focus on what truly matters. He is not essential. I need to establish the boundaries that I may not cross and beyond which no one is invited. I am glad Callie did not hear me. I carry my shame inside.

22

Two weeks after my discharge from Mass General, we moved from Beacon Hill back to our apartment, with the support of a visiting nurse. After caring for too many lonely geriatric patients suffering from dementia, she was visibly pleased to visit a woman her own age.

Or perhaps I was able to see her needs with more dimension than those of my MGH caretakers.

She came through the blistering heat to check my blood pressure, temperature, and swelling—dressed practically in shorts and sandals, her backpack of instruments damp against her T-shirt. I was grateful to her and reassured by my steady readings. But a pattern soon developed: she would talk to me about her life, staying much too long. Sensing her loneliness, I chatted encouragingly. I believed that I had my heart's full strength, just as an amputee feels as though his leg is still there. But in reality half my heart was dead, and I was working my way back to half the strength, half the immune system, and half the patience for others that had once been mine to give freely. Eventually, I used the old trick of standing up and letting my nurse talk as we meandered to the door. Once there, she discovered on her own that it was time to go. I would sleep an hour afterward, exhausted from trying to care.

After only one week in our apartment, we decided to put it on the market. Without the proximity of MGH and the fun, distracting, communal life with Juliana and Mark, we were too isolated. Our small apartment had served us well; it had been a cozy, simple base camp where we had packed and unpacked suitcases, frantically fulfilling our responsibilities to others. Now it was time for *us*, and Jack knew what we both needed: our feet planted firmly on spongy soil made of rotting pine needles.

Jack revved up his campaign for moving me to Maine. Marc and Torch would still be my doctors; Maine Medical Center, one of the top hospitals in the nation for cardiac care, would be my backup hospital and was forty minutes away. (Heck, it could take that long to get to Mass General from our apartment, depending on the traffic.) Our local hospital was five minutes up the road. The lake and my gardens would heal me; our Maine neighbors would watch over me; I would escape the summer heat that drained me; I could cook nourishing food in my big kitchen cooled by the breezes from Mount Washington; I could walk up and down our dirt road to the sound of rustling leaves, not screeching traffic.

Torch was beginning to come around. Marc didn't like the idea at all. They were both being sensible.

"Do you like this dress or this one?"

Jack is patiently watching as I flit from one outfit to another, indecisive as a hummingbird. He knows why I am nervous, and I am grateful that he is pretending not to notice; today we are going for our final hospital discharge meetings with Marc and Torch. I am trying very hard to look healthy and pretty for my doctors. If they say the word, I can move to Maine. Jack has already made a new work arrangement with Henri: he will spend four days a week in Boston, drive back to Maine on Thursday nights, and work from home on Friday. Callie has already made a schedule of friends and family who will move in when Jack is not there—to monitor me and enjoy a little vacation.

I have not primped like this since the ninth grade dances, when it seemed that absurd amounts of attention to appearance really did make a difference. I am giddy. In truth, I know that the dress is hanging off me and that my shoulders look like bent wire coat hangers. I've had my hair trimmed, but it has visibly thinned and there are streaks of gray in places I swear didn't have any before. I fuss with necklaces to disguise the mountain range on my chest, as if it matters. When I am done, I still look hollow-eyed, but the exaggerated ritual of dressing assures me that I did my best. I only have this one body, and it will have to do.

We walk into the hospital. This time I can make my entrance without a wheelchair. I'm up to one shaky twenty-minute walk a day. I cling to Jack's arm, and then I feel the terror flooding me again. My first walk in a crowd is a new and unpleasant experience. Without the protection of my johnny, no one knows that I am weak and can topple in a second. It feels as though we are in our own tippy little canoe on a fast-running river that splits and then joins around us. Jack is uncomfortable, too, realizing our mistake in not using a wheelchair.

Just then, a man walks swiftly into my back. He gets as far as my calf and realizes that there is a person under him and that he is breathing into her neck. He jerks around us, tosses off an apology, and keeps walking, a cell phone glued to his ear, blue blazer flapping, snappy briefcase knocking against his thigh. I watch him disappear into the crowd, blow-dried hair bouncing above other people's heads. Jack sees that I am sinking and we seek safety against the wall. *Is my heart racing dangerously? Did that man's cell phone deactivate the box? How badly will my leg bruise because of the Coumadin? When is a bruise a dangerous hematoma?*

"Love, let's get you a wheelchair."

"No," I say. "No, I can do this. I have to get used to it. Just give me a minute."

Once I was able to slug it out on the pavement with oblivious, rude people, to compete with the most aggressive for a place in the rush. After only one month in the land of the sick, it is already inconceivable how I survived daily in the kingdom of the well.

Marc shows no sign of noticing my dress, and putting on a johnny is deflating. In the tiny changing room, I am Cinderella returning to her rags after the ball—foolish to have forgotten my true status: Marc is my doctor and I am very sick. He pulls me into a safe, sober place of routine prodding, running through all the checks so familiar to me.

He says that my chances of another heart attack are "highly unlikely," that the greatest immediate danger is another arrhythmia, which would cause my box to go off. I must listen to my body and know when it is coming; my greatest risk is hurting myself when I pass out. I have only a second to drop to the ground, where I will be safest. Oddly, this is great news. I put an X through "heart attack risk?" in my notebook.

Reluctantly, he approves my move to Maine, pleased that I will have round-the-clock companionship. We'll see how it goes, he says, making clear that the real permission must be given by Torch, who is responsible for my care until he releases me today. I stretch up to hug Marc, and he blushes, as usual.

One down, one to go. In the elevator I ask Jack if he thinks that Marc was secretly pleased with my progress, if he thought I looked pretty.

Jack takes me to the cafeteria for lunch. It is an exorcism for him, a triumphant return to the days when I was fed intravenously and he tasted nothing. He gives me a tour, like a proud graduating senior showing a parent his college dormitory. The chairs and tables rise up to greet him. Stacks of glistening dishes stand on their ends and twirl. I see none of it. This was Jack's world. He deftly assembles my lunch on a plastic tray. I am amazed at the ballet of hungry people weaving in and out from each other while balancing trays. We sit in a corner and barely speak.

With time to spare before our meeting with Torch, I convince Jack to take me to Ellison 8. He clearly does not want to go there. This cafeteria has been quite enough, thank you very much. I march ahead, and when I totter he holds me up.

Once again I sway in the breeze of Ellison-8's sealed corridor, smiling at the main desk. It is a calm yet intense place. People look up after a while and then back at their work, eyes riveted to reports or beeping monitors. I am thrilled that their eyes do not recognize me. I see Stan poring over a patient's chart. Even without his mask, he looks like Groucho Marx. But Stan looks at me blankly as I approach him.

"You don't even know who I am, do you?"

He stares at me for a moment, then beams. Smiles burst like firecrackers around the desk. They marvel at me in a dress, at me standing up, at the color in my cheeks. (I've applied makeup carefully so they can't tell how pale I really am, ha, ha!) I am so proud to show them that their efforts were worth it and appreciated.

Stan offers to walk us to Torch's office in the Bullfinch Building. He presses the elevator button and the doors whoosh open. Everything slows down. In the center of the packed elevator stands a green giant in booties, cap, and dangling mask who has just left cardiac surgery, where he saved another person's life. He rides the elevator and walks the corridors with no more fanfare than I used to after leaving some everyday meeting.

"Torch," I breathe.

He stares. I look vaguely familiar. Mentally, he is still in the OR. Then he sees me.

"Get in here," he says quietly, and motions with a finger that could either mean get into the elevator or come in for a hug. I choose both, a magnet drawn to steel, unable to resist this primal feeling. He stares at the ceiling, appalled.

"Torch, you're actually blushing," announces Stan.

People in the elevator smile happily, like passersby who witness a bride and groom kissing after the wedding. The hospital employees know who this man is and who I must be.

I am perspiring and the smell is truly vile. I am horrified that the sweats can still be so violent. I pull away and want to apologize to the whole elevator. Maybe they don't notice, but the doors can't open fast enough for me.

I struggle to hide my difficulty in keeping up with Torch's relaxed stride into the Bullfinch Building. Our feet click and echo on the polished black stone floors. I came this way before on a gurney to have the box implanted, but all I saw were the delicate brass lanterns on the vaulted ceilings.

Torch excuses himself to change and to gulp his lunch—just plain turkey on whole wheat and a Coke. It is 4 P.M. and Kathy has had it ready for him since eleven.

He squeezes my ankles and listens to my heart and lungs. He examines the incisions. Then he gets to the part of the exam that clearly troubles him.

"Deborah, I want you to answer me truthfully. How is your brain?"

I think he is joking. He is not.

"Can you concentrate and for how long? What is your reading retention? How is your focus? I realize that the intellect is an important part of who you are, so be very honest with me."

These questions linger powerfully for Torch because no one knows exactly how long my brain was without oxygen when the left ventricle failed me.

I tell him of waking in Ellison-8 to nagging memories of where I was in a good book before my heart attack and wanting to finish it. How I had devoured that book and several others since. I tell him about remembering that Costa Rica is not an island and about my trip to Paris with the Haitian cleaning lady. I tell him about making vichyssoise by heart and then change that to "half a heart." He doesn't laugh. I also tell him that my vocabulary sometimes gets stuck—like the day I struggled to remember the word for doorknob. But it eventually came. Torch looks relieved.

Jack assures him that my only lapses of memory are when I call him Harry in the middle of the night. Torch gives a little chuckle. Then I ask him the same question that I asked Marc, the test question. His answer will determine how confidently I put one foot in front of the other.

"What is the likelihood of my having another heart attack?"

"Extremely remote," he says without hesitation.

I am amused at the contrast between the visual language of the surgeon ("extremely remote") and the language of probability used by Marc-the-cardiologist ("highly unlikely"). For the first time I grasp how their disciplines and personalities complement each other, how they work as a team.

"We still don't know exactly what caused this to happen in you, Deborah. You do not fit the profile. You don't have Marfan's syndrome nor do you show any arterial weakness that would cause your artery to spontaneously dissect. You don't have blood that coagulates unusually to create a clot. You had no plaque in your arteries. You are our mystery and our miracle. So the next time I should see you is in eight to ten years when we redo your bypass."

Whoa. No one said anything about this!

My eyes widen and fear flies out of me like bats. *You mean I have to go through all this again?* Torch sees that Jack is looking even more stunned than me and addresses him first, because they're the ones who struck a midnight deal when I was a chipmunk in a glowing burrow.

"You've always known this, Jack. Remember the family meeting?" Torch pauses for Jack to go there again. "But who knows what a redo will look like by then? With medical advances, I may be giving Deborah a pill." Torch shrugs.

Once again he works his magic. A pill. I've gotten very good at taking pills.

At the last minute I shyly ask him about sex, and Jack looks even more uncomfortable than he did a minute before. But I know he wants to know, too, even though sex hasn't interested either of us since May 12. Even now, the question has nothing to do with desire on my part—the drugs have destroyed that. It has more to do with trust in tomorrow. Sex has become a symbol rather than a goal.

"Sex is fine when you can walk up two flights of stairs with no breathlessness," Torch says, confirming the physical therapist's prescription. Jack perks up. I am still breathless on one flight of stairs, but less so.

Giving me yet another list of things to monitor—and making me promise to live with no lifting, no pushing, no pulling, no bending, no reaching, no ignoring even the smallest feeling in my body, no swimming and no putting cream or vitamin E on my scars until they are completely healed—he approves the move to Maine. Jack twinkles. I vow to Torch that he will see an even stronger woman the next time he examines me.

He says softly, knowing that tone communicates more than words, "You are welcome to come visit me as much as you like, Deborah. But at this point, I am no longer your doctor. Marc takes over fully now. You don't need a surgeon anymore. You don't need me. Of course, I will follow everything about your case. But Marc's in charge."

I wish all my old boyfriends had had his finesse. I feel a twinge of rejection anyway. I also realize that moving on is a good sign. It means that Torch's job is done. I have to heal the wounds that have bound us, by myself.

23

I AM LAID OUT in the backseat of the car like a garment bag. Jack has pillows behind my head, under my knees, propping up my feet. He slams the door and rounds the car to the driver's side with the excited step of a pioneer checking the hitches of his wagon. I must walk for ten minutes every hour, so we note the exact moment of our departure. Three times on 95 North—at a gas station, a state liquor store, a rest area—he eases me out of the car, takes my arm, and walks me. Each ten-minute interval is a long, self-conscious time. Do people notice that I am pale and my chest is concave or do I look normal? Do they think I am drunk or can they tell I am on drugs that make me dizzy? Do they notice that I am still marching back and forth even after they've finished walking their dogs and turned the ignition key?

No matter what others think, we are happy, purely happy. This car is our bubble and we pretend we are on a normal commute to Maine. But on the seat beside Jack is The Big Guy's book of custom maps, detailing every hospital location from every exit all the way home. Each ramp that we pass offers relief. *Whew—didn't have an arrhythmia yet, didn't need to use that one.* How long will this good luck last?

After three hours on the road, passing through Massachusetts, New Hampshire, and into Maine, I sit up as we drive down our little town's Main Street, where life is going on as usual. There's Jeff rearranging the carts at the grocery store, a pencil behind his ear. I wonder if there have been any shipments of parsley without my cajoling. (In a small Maine grocery store, parsley is an exotic. When I had to tell the teenagers at the checkout counter what it was, I felt sad for a whole generation.) Farther down Main Street is Reny's, Maine's small department store, where you can buy Woolrich shirt seconds, extra-extra-large overalls, frilly dresses for little girls, macadamia nuts, and off-register wrapping paper for 99 cents a roll. Women are marching in and out with the determination of the hunters who light up the town with orange jackets in fall. And there's Perri at the desk behind the large picture window of the bookstore, wittily and crankily giving a customer brilliant reading advice.

Finally we turn down our dirt road and drive out to the lake, as we did every week for eight years until I went to the hospital. Branches scrape the car and we lurch over the deep bumps carved by frost heaves and Mud Season. Peep frogs sing and mourning doves flutter away in a panic. Jack stills the motor and opens my door. The air is sweet with rain, freshly turned earth, pine needles—and silence, the soft, soothing silence of wind and water.

I enter our world in a trance. It is astonishingly as-it-always-was—constant as Jack, calming, unruffled by my approach as if to say, "Where've you been? Life is going on here!"

There is the green arbor with tulips at its base, in full bloom just as promised by the photograph Lucia sent a month ago when the tulips had barely poked through the winter's mulch. There is the glistening lake, which had sustained me with memories of its many moods. And there is the old Cape Hatteras knotted hammock in which I had imagined swinging softly to sleep when I needed to calm myself in the nuclear medicine lab.

Now here I am slowly folding up like a summer chair to kiss the ground. It is carpeted with white-pine seeds and they glow on the dark, moist earth like rust on an iron skillet. I notice for the first time, because I am a nose-length away, that the seeds are miniature versions of the pine cones dangling in the mature trees above. As my lips taste the earth and sap, I drink their promise of the restorative power of the seasons. I am home.

Then the tears come. It is June 27, 1997—my forty-fifth birthday. I've made it.

Sometimes you simply need to get through the bad part before you can cry hard. My brother and I once surprised dark, swirling things in the upper hayloft of a barn where we'd taken shelter from the rain. *Bats!* We screamed our way out of that barn and all the way home, peddling our bicycles as if life depended on it. But it wasn't until, soaked and shivering, we stowed our bikes in the garage that we began to cry hysterically, the kind of crying that sends you to bed with a headache.

Now that I was safe on our land in Maine, relief flooded me with tears. I would cry for the next year. These were unspecific, unscheduled tears—inspired by a kind word from a stranger, Jack's arm over me at night, the taste of a raspberry, my godson, Daniel, unconsciously twisting a stray hair behind my ear. Every day I was happy and sad at the same time, tears just behind the laughter, laughter quickly following the tears.

I now know that the flying black attackers of my youth were nothing more than barn swallows. Would all this turn out to be just as benign? When I moved back to Maine, there was only the terror that my heart would fail me and the box would fire. There was only the wondering about when this beautiful life would be snatched away again. I began to memorize everything so as to take it with me.

As word of my return went out, dusty cars and worn-out trucks bumped down our dirt driveway, and flowers filled the house. Friends tiptoed to the door, afraid of what they'd see. I was frail, and tinted a delicate shade of blue, but I was all there—and encouraged by their broad, surprised grins. Sally and Bob, our Maine switchboard, were the first to arrive in their old brown truck covered with bumper stickers. FREE TIBET. PEACE. NO NUKES. Bob's bottle-thick glasses were as misty as the shower stall he'd just left. His long beard was washed clean of sawdust for the occasion and his wet braid, tied neatly with rawhide, made a dark circle on the back of his shirt. Sally pulled me into her ample bosom, wrapping me in her pillowy body. And we sobbed. Her embrace was as grounding as the first hug she had ever given me—when I had stepped out from behind Jack with nervous embarrassment, the new Mrs. Heffernan, and Sally had whispered into my ear, "You've always been here."

One morning soon after our arrival, I woke to find the lake slick with pollen the color of unripe lemons. A week later, strong winds washed the pollen out of the cove. I watched it go in one mass, like a yellow sheet blown from the clothesline, carried by the current to the dam below. I am sure it does this every year, but I had never actually seen it happen. Before my heart attack, I might have seen the pollen floating in the cove; I might have noticed that it was suddenly gone. But in between I would have been at work and missed the parade.

In my new greedy joy, the parade was all for me; the yellow pollen was confetti, the russet pine seeds my red carpet. They dazzled me with their fecundity; life was renewing itself right under my uncertain bare feet. The silent, spectacular sunsets over Mount Washington—visible thirty miles away as the crow flies and crowning the far end of the lake—were daily proof of life's cycles. And in the dark of night, on my many trips to the bathroom, there was the moon, peeking through different windows as it made its trajectory through the sky. I'd be afraid to sleep again, afraid that I would never wake up in the morning. And suddenly warm light would be on my eyelids, inviting them to open and see the day.

An image came to me one sunset as I sat on our old weathered bench: I saw the year ahead of me as a time line bent into the shape of a circle, the shape of the setting sun, the earth, the circumference of a tree. This reminded me of the idea in yoga that strength comes from rounding the muscles. That meant releasing muscles instead of clenching them when assuming a difficult pose—the exact opposite of the body's first instinct. It was just as my father had taught me: to steer into the skid rather than slamming on the brakes.

The rhythms of the natural world and the lessons drawn from it in the ancient practice of yoga made me feel very small and insignificant, but not alone. I was beginning to see that I was part of something. Sometimes I couldn't contain the urge to put my arms around the rough trunk of my favorite old tree to tell him that I was listening. I made sure no one was around to see.

24

OH, THE BLISS OF BEING NICE AND COOL from the breeze off the lake while I lie in our bed during an early July heat wave!

In reality, I am cool because the sweltering heat is not making it to my toes and fingers. I pull up the down comforter and curl my toes around the hot water bottle that Jack slipped into the bottom of the bed. He enfolds me in his arms as best he can, an awkward production given how sore I am and how afraid he is to hurt me. He is sticky with sweat. In every position I feel the box tug under my skin. If I roll onto my stomach, it pushes against my breastbone. If I sleep on my side, it pushes against the mattress and into my ribs. I wear a nightgown now because looking at my own body is as repulsive to me as touching the murky stuff at the bottom of the lake. Jack keeps telling me to take it off, that I am beautiful to him, that he is proud of the scars. I am not.

Once we have arranged ourselves, Jack falls promptly into an exhausted, deep sleep. I know I will break it soon with my tossing and turning. Even if I weren't waking every hour to pee, I would be waking every hour to his insistent, almost angry prodding to be sure that I am alive.

I lie awake interminably, assaulted by images of my life just before the heart attack and in the hospital. The images insist that I review them continually but reveal nothing in return. I try to turn them off or switch to images of happier times as I once switched imaginary radio stations in my morphine-drunk head, but it doesn't work. Though Jack is lying close enough to me to feel like we have one skin, when the house is dark and quiet, I am all alone.

Dad once told my seven-year-old-sister, Ann, who was terrified of the dentist, that he would take her to her appointment and wait for her just outside the door, but "You're the only one who can sit in the dentist's chair." Even though love is right beside me now, I am the one who is alone in the dentist's chair. I listen to the darkness, and a hoot owl laughs.

Jack stayed in Maine for two weeks. He watched me become a six-year-old, ecstatic to see her friends drive up in an orange Volkswagen bus filled with plants and tools. Lucia gave me small things to do while her crew took charge. I potted pansies happily, slowly realizing her clever strategy: so long as my hands were dirty I did not miss the digging, the rearranging, the lowering of new perennials into their places that had been my spring ritual, a pleasure so deep that I never noticed the midges swirling and biting. We have a photograph from that summer day of me shielded by a hat, my thin, pale arms digging pathetically with a trowel. At the time, I felt strong as a prizefighter, though. I remembered my struggle to wield a pencil.

The loss of spontaneity was the most devastating thing during this period of adjustment. My every move had to be calculated—and I do not have a calculating bone in my body. A catastrophic heart attack destroys trust. No longer can you depend on sunrise following darkness; each second could be your last. Freedom gives' way to apprehension. You realize that you will never walk with nonchalance again; each push of your foot through the air seems the most astonishing piece of luck. And it is the same for anyone who loves you.

Jack supervised my ongoing retraining: learning not to lift anything, to ask for help, to pause after standing up and before taking a step. Jack saw my confusion and frustration when Sharon, the friend whose embrace had saved his life when he'd first arrived at MGH, knocked on the door and I could not rise to embrace her.

And I watched Jack tighten up. I saw him jump at my every sound and movement, his body tense with adrenaline, coiled for whatever it would take to keep me alive. When I asked him what he felt like, he conjured up the most horrible image he knows: a house overrun with mice. Here is a man who has no problem hanging off vertical cliffs, but who makes me sing "Jingle Bells" to scare away any mice and bats before he goes into the attic.

Now he said to me: "My life is like a mousetrap since you got sick. I set them all over our house and wait for them to spring—in the basement, in the kitchen, in the attic, in my bedroom, in my own bed."

I died again and again every time I saw that watchful, hunted look in those warm brown eyes that used to tilt with laughter. I hated myself for what I had done to him.

We tried and failed to make love. Our hunger to be together in the old ways, for the reassurance and renewal it always brought, drove us to try too soon. I dissolved into tears and he was pale with remorse, frozen above me in a push-up. "It's okay, baby. We have time," he murmured. We fell asleep holding hands, our other way of making love.

Well-meaning people often commented on how tragedy can transform relationships, making individuals appreciate life and each other more. We nodded politely but felt a tad irritated. Or perhaps we were jealous, deep down, because we had been taught this lesson as children, with the loss of my mother through death and Jack's father through alcoholism. We knew the importance of celebrating life's gifts, no matter how small. This habit had drawn us to each other in the first place, and saved us now. We celebrated everything, from my first solo trip to the toilet to Jack's first full day at work. We even celebrated trying to make love when the pills were killing desire and terror finished off whatever was left.

No, we could not love each other more than we already did, but our relationship was tighter because a third party, Death, had squeezed in. It lay in bed between us, making sleep feel like wasted time. It obliterated any feeling of innocence in our marriage. We had imagined that we were immune to betrayal, but death betrayed us. Finally we understood that one of us could leave the other and not come back.

The main difference between Before and After was that I now saw

132

my own death as a reality more certain than the sound of a slammed door, the sight of lightning splitting the sky, the bell ringing at the end of a school exam. I'd had a preview. This personal knowledge of death's swift, wordless finality deepened my appreciation for explorers whose adventures turn wrong, for soldiers, policemen, doctors, and firemen who face the end of life daily.

25

LIL AND PEG ARE STANDING outside the door when I awake from my nap, dressed in matching pastel outfits and shifting nervously from foot to foot. I throw my skinny arms around them and we cry.

Five years earlier, during an exhausted fit at the laundry, Jack and I vowed that we'd had enough and would hire a housekeeper. We worked long hours all week, and cleaning and laundry were simply too much. If someone could just come every other week for a couple of hours to vacuum . . .

At that very moment, a pretty, small woman with short, permed curls was saying a bit loudly to a friend, "Oh, by the way, I quit my job to go into my own housecleaning business. Spread the word." We leaped on her.

Jack asked for references and Lil said she was a Christian. Thinking he'd missed something with his one deaf ear, a souvenir of the pulmonary edema, he said, "That's nice. So am I."

"Praise the Lord," she responded, smiling broadly.

He nodded, still confused. Lil became a fixture in our lives and was soon bringing her friend Peg to clean with her. They laughed like schoolgirls, bustling through the house and making it smell of fresh air and lemons. During the week while we were working, they'd meet in our kitchen for coffee. Or say prayers on the beach. How could we say no to a few extra blessings?

I grind coffee beans and make them the strong brew that they love. They carry the small tray that is too much for me and we head for our sandy beach. I tell them how immeasurably grateful we are that they took care of the house over the last seven weeks. I tell them that I felt their prayers and how much all the cards from their nationwide prayer circle of good Christian women meant to me. I tell them that Jack and I could barely keep track of all the people praying for us—Catholics, Fundamentalist Christians, Protestants, Jews, Muslims, Hindus, Buddhists . . ."

Peg interrupts me and looks stern. "Buddha is dead."

Oh, dear.

I'm glad she stopped me before I mentioned Tink and her Raiki group. I wonder if she knew about Bob and Sally's ecumenical ceremony on this very beach when I was like an autumn leaf clinging to a branch. How do I explain that I do not discriminate in the prayer department without hurting their feelings? I decide to think about this later and pour another cup of coffee for my earthly saviors. All are equal and welcome on our windy point.

Religion is big in western Maine, and I am still finding my way. When I was first out of the hospital, some people approached me with their faith with alarming enthusiasm. They meant well, but I became wary. "Praise the Lord" was said about all manner of good fortune and not just the stuff that God should attend to, in my opinion. I was invited to prayer groups, church medical-support groups, and to read religious tracts, and there was an urgency to some of these invitations that rankled me. I resented religions that believed theirs was The Way, and I resented those who believed I might be vulnerable to their influence now that I was sick and weak. One most-loved friend even went so far as to say, "We were all so afraid you would die without God." Having been raised Catholic, I had had quite enough of this proselytizing. I agreed with my devout father: religion and spiritual beliefs are very private and individual. Besides, I felt that my God and I had a very good relationship, thank you very much, whether you called him Harry or Buddha.

My recovery was not without spiritual seeking, however. Months later I would think deeply about my relationship with the eternal. But that summer I was putting all my energy into my earthly body.

* * *

Jack went to work setting up our safety network. He discussed an intercom system with our electrician friend Joe. He bought the latest cell phone models, one for my baby-sitters when they drove me around town in my tiny old car, one for his station wagon. Even when he walked down the dirt lane to fetch the mail, Jack wore the beeper that Dave, The Big Guy, had supplied. Bill, our local security expert who disappears during hunting season, rattled down the driveway one day with a great idea: an alarm I could wear on my wrist like a watch whenever I was alone in the house. One push of a button and the ambulance would appear. Sold. One morning the emergency medical team guys showed up in the ambulance for a tour of the house and property so they would know all the places to look for me. We ran a test and it worked. The whole thing was surreal, like preparing for a nuclear strike in grade school.

We met with my backup cardiologist at Maine Medical Center, a lean runner, and I registered for cardiac rehabilitation there in September. We met with a doctor at the local hospital so that if anything went wrong I would not arrive as an unknown. At the check-in desk, a kind woman wearing a shoelace printed with hearts around her neck, her ID card dangling from it, entered instructions from my doctors about weekly blood tests into the system. It was difficult to face having a needle in my arm in Maine, the one place I'd always felt safe from assault. I could feel the tears welling when she instructed me to tell the desk each time that I was a "standing order." This was not going away.

Jack's assistant, Judy, prepared a laminated list of emergency phone numbers to post near every phone in the house. Our life had moved beyond simply dialing 911. On the list were phone numbers for all my doctors (office, home, beeper), blood labs, drugstores, the local ambulance company, six family members, and others. After fiddling with the design to make it easy to read in a panic, Judy drew a big pink heart in the middle. No one was going to miss the purpose of this list if she could help it.

We confirmed the baby-sitters' schedule that Callie had arranged through September, beginning with my godson Daniel's mother, Pam. Next would come Jack's daughter Mary Kate, whose nursing training was an extra comfort. Local friends volunteered to drive me anywhere anytime. The first to sign up was my eighty-year-old neighbor, Olga. Funny, I had thought that one day I might be of help to her.

I donated money to the American Heart Association, subscribed to the *Harvard Heart Newsletter,* and ordered a Medic Alert bracelet. The bracelet seemed to me a ghoulish bauble, and I took a long time to decide among the various styles. Finally I settled on a delicate ten-karat gold-filled chain with the Medic Alert medallion in the center. I would pretend it was jewelry instead of a dog tag. When it arrived with my emergency numbers and medicines etched into the back, I reluctantly fastened it to my left wrist—a golden handcuff that would never come off. I dangled it in front of Jack flirtatiously, but he looked at my face and wept.

As we swiftly constructed a world of support, we began to see that our new life was do-able in spite of the terror. I even learned that one of the registrars at the local hospital had a husband with frequent bouts of ventricular tachycardia and an ICD. When she told me that his box fired one time when he was riding his snowmobile, knocking him clear off while the machine proceeded, riderless, I didn't know whether to cry or cheer.

Then the two weeks of reentry were over and Jack had to return to work. He had gotten no rest. We counted the days until his return in our private math: Monday didn't count as a day of separation because we would have the early morning hours together before he drove to Boston, and on Thursday he drove north again, arriving in time for supper. That meant we were only apart Tuesday and Wednesday.

As Jack drove away, could my friend Pam feel the tidal tug between us? I waved long after he was gone. He called us six times before he reached Boston.

26

My days began to acquire a rhythm. I woke up around nine from a few stingy hours of sleep that didn't begin until 4 A.M. That was still more consecutive hours of sleep than I ever had in the hospital.

Upon opening my eyes, I would listen to the birds and smile woozily. Then I'd see the box of pills beside me and the horror would come flooding back. I'd gulp down my drugs and listen to my body. How irregular was my heartbeat? Where was I sore? Could I get up or was I too weak? Would the box go off? How much time did I have to make it to the toilet before the diuretics did their work? The incision on my right inner thigh burned when I sat up.

After peeing, I weighed myself to monitor weight gain due to swelling. I continued to decline from my original 142 and was now hovering at 129 pounds. At five-foot eight, my ideal weight was about 135, so I was getting very skinny. I recorded my daily weight in the journal my sisters had given me. It represented more than a system for monitoring my health; it was also a way to manage my confusion. My whole new life was in that book the way it used to be in my Day-Timer. My calendar was the box of pills; I knew what day it was by the empty compartments. I even took off my old watch and let the battery wear down. This sometimes meant that I was an hour off in taking my drugs, but the liberation from a conventional schedule was more important. I no longer marked the time the way other people did. I no longer raced against it.

I dedicated myself to walking in the morning—twenty minutes up and down our causeway while my energy was good and the air was cool, and sometimes again in the afternoon after my nap. Breakfast and lunch included more protein and calcium than before, on the advice of the MGH nutritionist. My baby-sitters and I feasted on Middle Eastern and Mediterranean concoctions I made from beans of every color and shape, yogurt cheese rolled in spices, fish cakes made with last night's poached salmon. I ate small portions several times throughout the day. Preparing food anchored me; there was life if I could mince garlic and sauté onions—as long as someone else did the dishes. Just after lunch, I would collapse with exhaustion and nap for two or three hours, the deep sleep that eluded me at night. I was still on hospital hours, sleeping better during the day. I awoke from my nap refreshed enough to enjoy preparing and eating dinner. By eight I'd be exhausted and by nine I'd be tossing and turning.

* * *

"No she is *not* all better. She will *never* be better!"

Mary Kate is hissing into the phone as I come into the kitchen after my nap. She slams the phone down and sees me. Her eyes dart away at being caught in an admission that only an outsider could have extracted. I accept her passionate defense of me against phone-invasion and try not to read too much into it. Our week together at the lake has been delightful for both of us—I think, I hope. I am pleased to have Mary Kate with me, for her nursing skill and her fun companionship. I am also trying not to let myself be too vulnerable with Jack's charismatic eldest in case this doesn't last, trying hard not to set my heart up for disappointment. Instead, I'm falling in love.

When I was in the hospital, Mary Kate and her husband, Walter, brought Jack back to our apartment to spend the night as an "exorcism." When Jack went into the guest room to kiss them goodnight, she turned to him as casually as if they were sharing a sandwich on a day-hike and said, "Dad, Walter and I have a lot to learn about love from you and Deborah." It was her first acknowledgment of our marriage as an intimate place, and it was a stunner. Our wise friend Bob once said, one muddy boot resting on the bumper of his truck, "Kids never learn the things you think you are teaching them. They learn from how you lead your life." Now here is Mary Kate in our kitchen, the first to volunteer to care for me, acting very much like Jack: choosing to see what is possible, not what is past.

"That was some insurance person. Your bill is overdue. She was annoyed that you were sleeping. She kept insisting that she'd heard you were better and that it would only take a minute. She wanted me to wake you up." Mary Kate is near tears.

I feel a tug. *Well, maybe I am just fine if I am walking into this kitchen. Maybe I am being a hypochondriac. Maybe it's not necessary, all this rest.* Having been unconscious through all the gruesome parts has left the entire event open to doubt. I feel guilty for not having paid a bill.

I look at beautiful, lanky Mary Kate, who has come to protect me from the outside world, at least for this one week. At thirty-five she suffers from early rheumatoid arthritis, a painful degenerative disease that she fights through to care for her young family. She knows what it feels like to be weak, what it feels like not to be able to imagine your future.

I pull down a few cookbooks for inspiration in feeding her well, wanting to pamper this mother of four who could not take care of her own fatigue until she came to care for me. We'll go to Turkey tonight. Stuffed eggplant and a fluffy fattoush salad. Watching my fierce, bony assistant move about the kitchen, I see us trying to walk up a small incline on the road this morning, my first attempt to go beyond the driveway and up a mountain. I was discouraged and breathing heavily.

"It's just like hiking, Deborah," Mary Kate said. "Remember how you used to slow and adjust your pace to the altitude? This is the same thing."

I remember. I can do that.

The effect of those few words was monumental. She flipped my feelings of humiliation into feelings of excitement at the prospect of beginning hill training. And my misgivings vanished, replaced by the belief that she really wanted me to be well, that what I was feeling with her was real.

During a visit the winter before, on a day when her rheumatoid arthritis was bad, I found Mary Kate straddling our big tub, weeping, unable to get in or out. Then she leaned on me. We have seen each other at our worst. Does that finally make us family?

27

TONI KNEADS MY COLD FEET, soft and squishy from disuse. Thank heavens Torch finally said that my scars were healed and I could have a massage. Toni says nothing, just sighs a little. The oil is warm and velvety as she leans into my calves with long strokes. She knows to go carefully because of bruising due to the blood thinners. I yearn to relax like Raggedy Ann, but I am brittle as a china doll. I remember how dry and itchy my stick-legs were in the hospital, how I melted when Eric-the-floating-green-shirt massaged my feet once with lotion when I couldn't sleep from the cramps and we got in a little trouble for it afterwards. *No oil near the scars.*

We are in a small room off the back of the never-finished house that Toni's husband built in a field ringed with views of distant hills. This warm room has always been a cocoon for me. I surrender to her.

My whole body sighs as Toni works her magic. She does not flinch at how ugly it is now, slashed and bubbled where there was once smooth white skin. She begins at the lower end of the scar on my right thigh and concentratedly massages every ripple in the seam. It is creepy, giving me a metallic taste in the back of my mouth.

"I have to do this, Deb." Her voice is low, almost a whisper. "Your nerve endings and muscles will attach faster, the scar will fade faster, and you'll have less scar tissue. It's important to touch the wounds so they heal."

As always with Toni, it sounds as though she is talking about more than just my body. I have not been able to bring myself to touch my scars, so the pressure of her fingers is triggering tears of recognition. As I come back to life, my inner body speaks with these saline spills the way a spring beneath the earth bubbles up to tell of hidden pools of vitality.

Toni gently rubs oil into the scar on my chest and I look away, repulsed. The skin stretched over my box itches insanely. When she rolls me over, we have to stuff a soft pillow under my left shoulder to elevate the box so I don't feel it. With her hands, she pushes away the numbness, the hospital-bed memories trapped in my back and buttocks, inviting them to wake up, to feel again. As she coaxes my body to relax, I realize that I have been in more discomfort from the pretzel I have become than from the incisions.

"You need to see my friend Judy Shedd, a cranial osteopath," she says. "You need the both of us to bring back your alignment and circulation. She's good. Tell her I sent you."

Dr. Judy Shedd, D.O., the sign reads outside a white clapboard building hung with nasturtiums and impatiens. To become a D.O., doctor of osteopathy, one takes premed courses in college and then goes through four years of medical school for osteopathy. I looked up osteopathy in my dictionary in preparation for this first meeting. "A medical theory that emphasizes manipulative techniques for correcting somatic abnormalities thought to cause disease and inhibit recovery," the entry read. *Inhibit recovery*. I definitely do not want to inhibit recovery. I want to cheer it on! Hio! Then I looked at its roots, *osteo:* "bones, from the Greek." And at the definition of *somatic:* "of or pertaining to the wall of the body cavity, especially as distinguished from the head, limbs, or viscera." *What?* All I know is that an osteopath relieved my father of his chronic back pain and that my back aches terribly. I cannot stand up straight and I long to stretch. I am at Judy's office on blind trust. Marc said that as long as I do nothing without his approval, I am allowed to explore body work if it makes me feel good. He approves of cranial osteopathy.

Giggles float out of the treatment room, and behind them Dr. Shedd, in a floor-length dress, all five feet of her, with a halo of messy pale-blond hair streaked with just enough telltale white to balance the giggles.

"Come on in," she sings, and I obey. I have since learned that Judy lives for music and that her voice is just another way that she consorts with the angels.

I lie on my back and she holds my head, making swift prodding motions. Then she goes to work on my spine with her eyes closed, rhythmically pushing it here and there. She puts on a rubber finger, opens my mouth, and sticks her finger in and out before I can bite it.

"Yeow!"

"Got it." She smiles pleasantly and I reel from the twanging pain in the back of my mouth.

"What the hell did you do?"

"Oh, your palatine was out. Probably from the intubation. I just put it back into place," she hums. "Feel-better now?"

I do. Ripples flow from my head through my body. Something has been put right.

"Can you go swimming?"

"You mean 'right now' or at all?"

"Both."

"My scars are healed, so I can go in the water now. And my doctors say I may swim eventually when I have the strength and if someone swims right beside me, because if the box goes off, I could drown."

I am a skinny-dipper and a water rat, so I am devastated by the idea of never swimming freely again. I think back to my family's tradition of swimming and how we especially loved to swim in the rain. We had the town pool all to ourselves—no bullies, no tans, just six pale children who could swim like fish. I come back to the room and Judy is talking as though I've never left.

"I thought so. It's just that I'd really like to get you in the water after my treatments. Floating would be good for you."

She pauses, thinking, then asks, "Do you have any noodles?"

I think about the contents of my larder and count the bags of pasta stored there. "Sure, lots of 'em. Do you mean specifically egg noodles?"

Champagne bubbles fill the room as her giggles turn into whoops. I join in, it feels so good. But I have no idea why we are laughing. It is simply infectious and we are having a fine, riotous time. I haven't laughed like this in months.

"I don't mean *food!* I mean *noodles*—those bright-colored plastic tubes that children play with in the water. You know what I mean. You can float on them." She cannot stop laughing.

I have no idea what she is talking about. But I vow to buy a pair and float on them as instructed. I'll do anything but take more pills.

As I leave the office, I notice a battered black leather bag like the one Dr. Cohen used to bring to our house when we all had the flu and Mother was beside herself.

"My father's. He was a doctor, too."

Jack is looking at me nervously—with consent in his eyes, apprehension in his body. I move into the water with two fluorescent tubes, the prescribed noodles. I hook my arms over the pink one like a touring president in the backseat of a car. Then I struggle to lift my legs off the sandy bottom and over the green one, positioning it behind my knees.

The edges of my mouth slowly curve up to touch the overhanging branches of maple trees. Here I am, floating in fresh, cool lake water perfumed with the tinny smell of fish and bugs. Jack is crying and I am swimming in my own new way. This is even better than swimming in the rain.

* * *

I have since learned that Judy Shedd is considered a major talent in cranial osteopathy. Dr. Andrew Weil's book *Spontaneous Healing* gives a good explanation of the field. Cranial osteopathy is a system founded by Dr. Andrew Taylor Still in 1874. His idea was to adjust the body mechanically to allow the circulatory and nervous systems to function smoothly, bringing natural healing power to any ailing part. The head was key. He found that its cranial sutures (joints linking the twenty-six bones of the skull) move in a way that resembles breathing, mirroring the rhythmic expansion and contraction of the central nervous system and vital organs—the very ones working overtime for me now that half my heart's power was gone. Feeling the head for its breathing pattern can therefore pinpoint blockages in the body that can lead to disease. The main cause of impairment of the system is trauma, and trauma can begin at birth. If the first breath of life is not perfectly full, the theory goes, the cranial rhythms are restricted from the start. In prodding my head and body, Judy was feeling for blockages and attempting to open them—inviting the natural healing power of my body to go to work unrestricted.

It was, and continues to be, important for me to actively participate in my recovery beyond following a prescription of allopathic medicine, rest, and exercise. So I designed my own complementary medicine plan, and was delighted to find my fumblings corroborated by renowned heart surgeon Dr. Mehmet Oz in his book *Healing from the Heart*. Each week I went for a massage or cranial osteopathy appointment. Under Toni's and Judy's care, the frost that permeated my body slowly thawed. I began to believe in the day when I would be able to stand straight, when my shoulders would uncurl and I would breathe deeply. I dared to fantasize about a full, uninhibited body stretch with the entitled looseness of a cat.

28

THERE IS A LUMP IN MY LEFT BREAST. Barely perceptible, but there absolutely. I keep pressing the spot lightly, hoping that it is my imagination. But Jack found it. I have a witness.

My friend Cynthia is here for a few days to take care of me, and will drive me to my appointment with Dr. Dixie Mills, a breast surgeon who saw me a couple of times in Boston. She has since moved to the Maine coast to work for Women to Women, a practice founded by Dr. Christiane Northrup, M.D., a pioneer in women's health care.

I am on a doctor's examination table again. I can handle this. I really can. I know the drill. I put on a johnny without instructions. I place my hands behind my head as though it's a lazy Saturday afternoon and I haven't a care in the world. I lie still, breathe, focus on the positive. But I turn my head away from Dixie as she leans over me with her pale, pretty face and red lipstick. She begins to knead the right breast gently, methodically. When will this end? A box in one breast and a lump in the other. I have been a good girl. Enough is enough.

Dixie finds the lump. Then she puts that warm jelly on the end of the ultrasound wand and goes slowly over the same area like someone searching thoroughly for coins on the beach. Finally, Dixie smiles a little and pulls the wand away, giving me a towel to clean my breast. I wipe at the goo absentmindedly. I am looking at her, riveted.

"It's a cyst. But let's watch this thing. It's too small to aspirate. If it's uncomfortable, let me know. It will probably just disappear on its own, like the others."

Friends and I joke that we wouldn't have breasts if it weren't for cysts, a nervous, macho joke, the humor of smoke jumpers. No matter how many times I have gone through this drill, it still takes my breath away until the doctor smiles. *Safe again.* To celebrate, Cynthia and I drive to a fancy coffee shop. I buy her an iced coffee and Jack a new car mug for his commute to Boston. I order juice. It may as well be champagne.

Next we head to Maine Medical Center so I can take a stress test in preparation for enrollment in the fall cardiac rehabilitation course. After running as fast as I can on the treadmill—with my ICD turned off, terrified of having an arrhythmia, panting and shaking—I collapse into four pairs of arms which lift me to a chair. I think I did pretty well, but the supervising doctor is uncomfortable with my questions and flees before I am done. Maybe somebody is dying. I try not to judge. They give me a cookie and juice.

I return to the waiting room utterly spent. It is crowded, and most of the people are elderly, though some only look old. Most are overweight. Their skin is ashen, their gazes vague, apprehensive. Some lean on their escorts. Some breathe heavily. I hear the gravely voices of lifelong smokers, a sound I've always liked. I look for Cynthia's long hennaed braid and magenta tunic and am surprised to see her textbooks closed on her lap. We met in 1978 during our graduate studies at Harvard, where we seemed to be the only ones working our way through school and shopping at Goodwill. Today she is a tenured professor of Indian art history at Middlebury College. But instead of preparing her lecture as planned, she is looking around the waiting room in a controlled panic, examining people the way I imagine she scrutinizes Hindu temples in the jungle.

Cynthia rises quickly when she sees me and jams her books into a battered old briefcase. We walk into the sunshine and she mumbles polite questions about the procedure until we are finally alone in the car. Then she turns to me.

"What are you doing here?" she screeches, as if I am a lost and naughty child, her eyes wild, searching mine as though I know the answer and am holding out on her. "What are you doing with these people? There must be some mistake."

The reality—easily disguised by nice meals and candlelight on a lake—has hit her. Seeing her reaction is oddly comforting; it reassures me that I am not crazy, that all this has really been quite a change in plans. I am glad to be reminded that in another time we hurtled through Cambridge at night on our beat-up bicycles with only narrow reflector ribbons tied around our chests and ankles as protection, powered by our strong young legs, lungs, and hearts.

Safely back in my corral on the lake after these brief forays into the world, I would turn to nature again for proof that some things are constant. Summer proceeded unperturbed and on good days I reveled in my sudden retirement. The season unfolded with warm, sunny days balanced by just enough rainy ones so I could sleep deeply. My husband and baby-sitters took away all practical concerns and I was lazy. For the first time since the endless summers under the pine trees of my childhood, I was completely in the season. Paying attention to summer became a form of meditation.

Our peninsula was like a nature conservancy. The blue heron arrived on schedule and stalked the shore for fish. Loons nested and wailed. The pair of mink that lived in the rocks on our shore hung out with me occasionally, bobbing in the water, sticking only their noses into the air to smell me sitting on the shady beach. My favorite annual ritual was the presentation of new mallard ducklings by their parents. One morning as I was twisting a honeysuckle vine into the arbor, I felt a light hammering sensation on my big toe. And there were the tiny yellow balls of feathers, insisting on the breakfast of bread crumbs their mother had promised them.

"Gardening is an instrument of grace," wrote May Sarton, and now our years of patiently removing hard-packed acid soil by the shovelful and digging in well-composted manure were showering us with grace. Flowers visited in an orderly annual sequence: pulmonaria and bergenia, lily of the valley, lamium, lady's mantle, forget-me-nots, bleeding hearts, peonies, irises, goatsbeard, coralbells of every sort, and steady waves of astilbes and lilies.

As for edibles, there was barely enough sun passing through our property to grow herbs. We planted herbs and cherry tomatoes in pots, which we moved around to chase the light. In the farm stands that summer, perhaps because of the long, cold spring, the fruits were spectacular—plump and glistening in green cardboard boxes. They revived my ailing taste buds, each fruit's season marking my progress. The strawberries ripened late and I ate them piggishly, well into the first half of July. The raspberries I ate delicately, one by one, or sometimes in desperate handfuls. Then peaches arrived and I enjoyed one juicy, golden orb each day. As the raspberries left us, wild blueberries took over, and my nephew Chris and I made blueberry-raspberry pancakes slathered with maple syrup from our local supplier. The blackberries were almost too beautiful to eat, dark perfection against the emerald green tiles in our kitchen. And soon there would be reddening apples in Gyger's orchard.

Still unable to do much more than swoon from postoperative fatigue, I spent many mornings swinging gently in the hammock strung over the huckleberry bushes, smelling them ripen against the spicy scent of pine sap. Or I might drift about the property inspecting plants for bugs. Sometimes I felt frisky and pulled weeds or dead-headed flowers for a few minutes. I made notes on future improvements and I dreamed of plunging a shovel—just a small one—into the earth all by myself. When Lucia and her crew came to do the heavy work for me, I followed her like a puppy.

29

I AM STANDING ON THE FRONT PORCH surveying freshly dug holes and scattered potted perennials, exhausted from a morning of watching Lucia's crew work. They make me feel like I have something to do with this year's plantings, though all I can do is point. They are packing up to go so I can have a quiet lunch and collapse into bed for the afternoon. It's amazing to me how tired I become from interaction. Lucia can read me like the onslaught of mildew on a begonia.

"Off to bed, Deborah."

She squints at me and gives me a hug around the shoulders. As I nestle in, we see a car pull down the driveway. A man gets out with a clipboard. He stands at the bottom of the stairs.

"Is one of you Mrs. Heffernan?"

I raise my hand, obedient to anyone who takes attendance.

"I'm from the state building-inspection office, and we understand you've done some renovation. I wanted to ask you a few questions."

A flame rises fast from the pit of my stomach into my throat and lodges there. I am in a panic. *How do I know he isn't lying? What does he really want? Jack is in Boston. I can't answer any questions by myself. What if I say the wrong thing?* My fatigue is acute, and he is one more thing than I can handle. Simple as that. I always had extra energy, a kick to handle just one more thing. All that is gone. This inspector is an invader. No one comes here anymore unless Jack says so. I am swiftly unraveling, and Lucia can see it in a flash.

"Could you come back another day?" she suggests nicely, her arm still around me.

No, he insists. He's come all the way from Augusta. *Then why didn't you make an appointment?* I want him to go away.

"I'm not well, you see." I try to explain, becoming jittery. "I can't talk to you. I am tired. My husband . . ."

He is unmoved. Lucia becomes defensive. "She's just had open-heart surgery. Please come back another time."

But he looks at me as though we are lying. After all, I am young and thin; my bluish pallor has receded and the summer sun has put a little color in my cheeks. I feel his impatience. I can see him thinking, *Of all the excuses I've heard, this is a good one.* His suspicion taps right into my own doubts that I am really sick, and I feel guilty.

Then he says, "I'd just like to look around."

"Look around? You said you wanted me to answer questions. Look around to your heart's content."

I look at Lucia with relief. He wanders around the corner where we put in some new windows. Then satisfied, he takes off. I am too upset for lunch and softly cry myself to sleep. A silly incident, really, but I feel violated. *I can't even handle a man with a clipboard. Where have I gone?*

To bed. And I liked it. An experienced inhabiter of her bed, Virginia Woolf observed that the ill prefer poetry to prose, and I was no different than the rest of the recumbent. That summer, in addition to my usual diet of literary fiction, I devoured poetry books that I had not opened since high school, underlining whole pages. My senses had been sharpened, and only poetry's compression captured the alert, immediate presence of the twilight in which I existed, somewhere between life and death.

With friends like Lucia in the garden and books piled high beside me, I did not care how I had gotten to bed. I was just happy to be there, happy to hand to my bed full responsibility for bearing the weight of my being. I was bone tired.

It was not until four years later, when I was writing this book—and after a few carefully challenging questions from my pal Juliana—that

I fully understood my relief in going to bed: I had been depressed, not just physically exhausted. It took me hours of struggle and reckoning before I could write that simple sentence, because I was a highly capable woman and depression was simply not in my vocabulary. It was a word used by people who were histrionic or installed in institutions dripping with ivy. Boy, was I wrong. While a little case of the flu can offer relief from having to perform in the world, anyone who prefers recovery from open-heart surgery to returning to the world is depressed.

Today, depression and anxiety are gaining in recognition and treatment as normal side-effects of heart disease, especially for those who have experienced a cardiac event, and most especially those who have undergone surgery. But during that first summer of recovery in Maine I had no idea that some degree of sadness is to be expected. Cozy and content in my personal nature conservancy, grateful to be alive and demonstrably loved, I was confused to notice that I was also sometimes moody, anxious, on edge, afraid, and despairing: depressed.

In November 2001, *The New York Times* reported that although there were no absolutely conclusive statistics about the incidence of depression after bypass surgery, it was estimated that from 30 to 75 percent of patients suffer from post-operative depression. There were several theories as to why depression can occur post-operatively, including the impact on brain chemistry of prolonged anesthesia (open-heart surgery typically lasts four or five hours), hypothermia (my body had been chilled to 32 degrees), and the heart-lung machine.

The theory that called out to me, though, was the impact of the patient's mind-set before the operation. Ambushed by the spontaneous dissection of my LAD, intubated without anesthesia, and then raced into emergency open-heart surgery, clearly my mind had not been at peace. It was in shock.

But neither had my mind been at peace when I left my office on the day of my astonishing MI. Work is where most of us spend most of our days, so it stands to reason that our feelings about our work can affect the state of our minds. In my case, what had begun as an exciting adventure in the world of business had become a relentless series of improvisations. I was worn out from pleasing too many clients in too many time zones, and from too many corporate cultures that kept changing during fourteen years of nonstop mergers, downsizings, reorganizations, and technological advances. There are consultants who thrive on continually justifying their existence, on beginning again and again without the continuity of old relationships, but I did not. I had mistaken being challenged and needed for personal satisfaction, becoming so good at the game that I even fooled myself. I was the child who climbs higher and higher into the tree and is suddenly stuck, with no idea how to get back down.

But it was another, more basic mistake that ultimately broke my spirit: a troubled relationship with the person I loved and admired most at my company, who did not place the same value on trust that I did. As a result, I was always on edge in my own office, unable to rest and recharge. Trust permits the high-wire act to continue; it is the wind under our wings, a refreshing deep sleep after a long, hard day, the very oxygen of partnership. How could I have worked for so many years without basic trust?

Like many people in the prime of their lives with multiple responsibilities, I was so busy "doing" that I had not noticed the danger signals, the signs that my life was losing coherence and context. By the time of my dissection, there were two people inhabiting my body: the one in Maine at my chopping board looking across a lake and the one in a boardroom looking at poker faces. Like most people, I needed to earn money in order to pay the bills, but if I'd been able to be really honest with myself, I would have recognized the ambivalence, the dangerous dissection in my soul.

Oh, it was easy to recognize the fracture in others, the ostensibly successful whizzing through revolving doors, beautifully dressed and imagining that no one can see the tension in their faces, in their necks and hands. I certainly never saw myself as "one of those people"; I had never totally surrendered my free spirit. Or, had I? I am ashamed to admit that I remember trying to cultivate the ponderous scowl that seemed to be ubiquitous on the faces of "serious" professionals. My giggle always rose, but suppression often won the battle.

My split in two was compounded by emotional exhaustion. My siblings and step-children were angry. For the most part it was well disguised, but it was there. And I understood. Anger is part of every family's story—misplaced anger that comes from sadness and grief, unexamined anger that undermines understanding and loads the simplest gift with buckshot. So I poured more compassion and generosity into everyone, all the while feeling increasingly isolated and despairing. Depleted. Yes, I had been both exhausted and sad well before my LAD dissected—despite my smiley competence and Jack's devotion. My metaphorical heart was fragile well before my physical heart broke.

An innovative leader in cardiac care and a proponent of total lifestyle change to reverse heart disease, Dean Ornish, M.D. found that in addition to obvious stressors like war or unemployment or caring for a child with a terminal disease, a "perception of isolation" can also put people in a chronic state of stress and compromise the immune system. Had my secret feelings of isolation from my family as well as in my work, exacted a toll on my health? In the year before my MI I had taken to arriving at meetings with a whole tissue box in my briefcase, because I was sick with yet another cold or flu. Was it responsibility or vanity that made me feel too busy or too essential to go to home and rest? Even on weekends, I was never, ever still. I had utterly lost my ability to recompose.

Like most busy people, I had no idea of the biological necessity of solid, regular breaks from pressure and performance—until my LAD dissected, threw me into bed, and forced me to face my life in order to save it. During summer afternoon nap-time, my bed became headquarters for tentative forays into reconsidering my life. There I began to examine everything that could have landed me in cardiac land, an excavation that turned out to be essential for rebuilding my mind-set. The data was persuasive. Five major investigations in the 1990s found that post-cardiac event patients who were depressed or socially isolated were two to five times more likely to die in the next six to twelve months after a heart attack. Though recumbent, I had vital work to do. I had been given time to face and resolve a few things and I was going to use it. Somehow I knew that my life depended on it.

Now no one could accuse me of being a wimp for hiding under the covers. Illness became both my protector and a weapon I could brandish, should anyone disturb the peace I needed for restoration.

With Jack as the fiercest defender of my privacy, I was responsible for no one and marching toward no deadline for the first time in many, many years. Though I was sad and bewildered, I relished being still and unoccupied. The languor of recovery reconnected me with my original self, with a childhood of spending afternoons alone in the woods, reading on a bed of moss. I was grateful for this happy memory, a life-saving gift from my parents. I knew that solitude was not the same thing as being alone. I did not chafe at stillness and sequestration, as some heart attack victims do. I loved it.

But I was afraid of dying alone. At any moment. Like now.

Once I was the kind of person who flew before dawn from Boston to meetings in Chicago, then drove across the northern plains of Indiana, chased by a dark storm, to make a meeting in Fort Wayne before flying back to Boston. If it was Friday, I'd change planes and land in Portland, often meeting Jack at the airport, after his plane flew in from another part of the world. Then the two of us would drive an hour to our old house on the shore of a small Maine lake. And think nothing of it. Now a trip to the hammock was dangerous. "The box" could fire at any time, leaving me flailing in the huckleberry bushes, if I managed not to hit a rock on the way down. Illness had stripped me of the armor that no one realizes we are wearing in the kingdom of the well. Now I was afraid of everything—a scaredy-cat instead of a bold road warrior. If Jack drove over 15 miles an hour on our way to the local hospital for blood tests, I cowered. I was safe only in our big old bed.

Feeling safe is essential to recovery from any illness, because every part of the patient's being is preoccupied with survival. In my case, guards were required. I needed others to supervise my reentry and help me recognize what was too much for me. Jack and babysitters established my schedule and boundaries so all my energy went into recovery. The schedule was posted on all doors and strictly enforced.

My sisters restrained their anxiety by taking turns as the daily caller, reporting to the others how I was doing; I spoke with Dad every evening, which was very good medicine for both of us. I was not allowed to answer the phone, and certain calls were never to reach me. All conversations had strict time limits because I could be oblivious to fatigue until it was too late. Many people thoughtfully wrote regular notes rather than calling or visiting so I would not have to use my precious lung power. I still spoke in a whisper.

My safe haven was in the wilds of western Maine. For other patients it might be the four walls of an apartment where visitors are buzzed in or left outside. The important thing is that your place of recovery allow you to rebuild your strength and confidence without distraction or criticism. It matters that you are surrounded only by people whom you love and trust. I am convinced that my chance of survival increased the minute the people I loved most showed up at the foot of my hospital bed. Love may have given my immune system a boost, too, because over the next few years with half of a functioning heart and overworked lungs, I was rarely sick with more than a case of the sniffles. I have learned that in illness as in life, the company you keep may be more important than the medications that you take.

30

SOON PLUMES OF GOLDENROD were crowded along the roadside, bringing both splendor and sneezes. I called Juliana and Mark to hear about their annual August family reunion. It had not been a good holiday. They'd gotten word that Mark's estranged brother had died, released from a life that had caged him.

Gracie the parrot had fled her cage, too. As the family walked down to the beach through a field, Gracie had taken flight into the first open space she had ever seen, launching straight off Juliana's shoulder like a rocket. They called her name desperately, but she would have none of it. She swooped and circled deliriously over the field, then disappeared into the surrounding forest. They split into groups and searched for hours. How long could a bird with clipped wings fly on instinct alone? They peppered the *Vineyard Gazette* with "Lost Parrot" ads, but no one found Gracie. There would be an occasional false parrot-sighting, just enough to get their hopes up. But as September approached, they accepted that Gracie was gone. Even if she had managed so far to survive the cats of Martha's Vineyard, she would never survive the winter, far from her native tropical habitat or her luxurious Boston cage.

"I've cried more over that damn bird than over my own brother's death," Mark said, incredulous. Our big, strong prince of a friend—who'd supported Jack through haunted hours, then lost the brother he loved—was finally able to fall apart. It was Gracie's last gift.

By late August, when Maine skies grumble threateningly from off-shore hurricanes, I felt the stirrings of anger. Getting sick had been sort of like running away when I was six and hiding behind the Big Rock in our front yard to find out if I was loved. But now that I had nearly died and was being fussed over, my elation at feeling loved was tempered by very real, ugly anger.

First, I blamed my job and the mine fields of corporate life. Then I focused on a friend turned client who had sabotaged a highly visible project and caused me weeks of anguish. I fought the urge to blame our families, but it was there nonetheless, itching, festering. I made a couple of vague attempts to talk, which they either missed or deliberately side-stepped. Too dangerous, too soon.

I blamed my body for having betrayed me. I reviewed the events leading up to my heart attack again and again, searching for causes. I read articles in health magazines and medical journals and peppered Marc with questions. Could I have caught a virus in Italy? Had he checked my homocysteine level? Was he *sure* that my blood did not tend to excessive coagulation or that I did not have Marfan's syndrome? Could yoga have done it? (At the last question, he erupted with laughter.)

Had I not exercised enough? Could that disgusting Big Mac I ate when I was faint with hunger in Detroit have done it? Why did I take everything so seriously, as though I could make a difference? Why hadn't I established stronger emotional boundaries? Could I have actually done this to myself? This was the worst anger of all.

Marc told me that I was doing very well from the eyebrows down, and that I had to stop puzzling over why and begin focusing on getting better. IT had happened and the time had come for acceptance. A clot and a torn LAD had done the damage. That was all they knew. Marc was right, but I couldn't stop the questions from assaulting me when I was enjoying sunlight through a beech leaf.

Jack, too, suffered from the tyranny of "why" beneath his competent surface, winding tighter and tighter into a ball of compressed emotion. Friends approached him in vain. Always he said he was fine-just-fine, while inside he was consumed with guilt. Had he not protected me enough? Was there a signal he missed? Should he have encouraged me to quit and move to Maine ahead of him? I saw the pain of self-recrimination in his eyes, in the set of his jaw. But he would wave me away, tears welling. Not now, not now.

I often thought about what would have happened on May 12 if I *had* quit my job after the last bout of near-pneumonia, if I *had* been living in Maine instead of sticking it out in the rat race for just a few more months as planned. Would the story have been different? Would I be pleasantly writing a cookbook now instead of this memoir?

No, I would be dead. Being minutes from MGH had saved my life. When I finally realized this, I squirmed into Jack's arms before he could climb out of the car, his arms already full of groceries. I told him the truth: *our* decision that I remain in my job for a few months longer, just minutes from him and MGH, had made all the difference in my fate. This was my first truly healing thought, a release for both of us. Over the next year, this fact always settled any doubts when I began to thrash emotionally, which was often in my search for *Why me?*

It was clear that just as my physical heart needed time and space to heal, so did my spiritual heart, and so I booked an appointment with a therapist in the fall, knowing I could not go where I needed to without help. My two hearts were the parallel wheels of the old station wagon that I'd steered into the skid when I was sixteen. Trying to heal both hearts would get me over the bridge now, even if my progress was in slow motion, like the day I skidded down a hill while the snow fell softly.

As the first maple leaf bled scarlet, the parade of baby-sitters came to an end. Although I treasured having friends, sisters, and Jack's daughters to myself for one whole week and getting to know each other all over again, I also wanted to savor the intimacies and insights of each visit rather than move immediately on to the next.

Having a variety of baby-sitters had been therapeutic. Each visitor wanted to hear every detail of my story, but worried that I was tired of repeating it. Far from it. These conversations helped me to believe it had all really happened and to fill in the gaps in my knowledge. In June, the shock of the words reverberated in my body and shook the terror loose until it fell out like stones for me to collect and examine later. By August the story had become more like a chant, bringing me closer and closer to acceptance. My life had changed irrevocably.

I wanted my privacy back. I had not been alone since May 12— me, the woman who once hopped on airplanes the way other people walk to the mailbox; who at twenty-two had moved to a tiny village in the Swiss Alps, not knowing a soul or the German language beyond "Where is the toilet?"; who had spent many years boyfriendless and penniless in her Cambridge apartment lighting a candle at a table set for one each night.

I wanted to think without interruption, to let my brave, cheery face fall, to acknowledge the sadness and anger that were lurking just below the gratitude. The assertion of my independent self was a sign that the terror was beginning a very slow retreat. If "the box" hadn't fired yet, maybe, just maybe, I could be alone for a little bit.

I began to look forward to my scheduled rest each afternoon because I could be alone to take stock. George Orwell, dying of tuberculosis, found that he could calm his panic by writing down, as a reporter might, the exact contents of the room around him. I, too, sought comfort in inventory. Surrounded by a mess of pillows I stared at the ceiling for hours. Water and light reflections rippled across it. Time floated by like lily pads, bobbing and suspended. I saw faces in the knots of the red-pine boards and remembered happily playing "I Spy" in bed with Great Aunt Dizzy as we stared at her swirling floral wallpaper, our cold little feet resting on her flannel nightgown. *There is a deer, an owl, an ugly man, a bird.*

My fantasy life was active as I stared blankly at the ceiling and furnishings. I imagined doing things for which I had no energy. It was rather like reading the book review instead of the book. After my rests,

I felt I had gone far and wide and accomplished great things. And this was sometimes true because, as Eudora Welty wrote, "A sheltered life can be a daring life as well, for all serious daring starts from within."

Twenty years earlier, I had crossed a turbulent North Sea from Sweden to England, lonely and terrified in my hard berth, fighting nausea valiantly. I was speeding to the next adventure and then returning home to my beginnings in Massachusetts. With each heave of the big ship, I thought I would die at the bottom of the sea. The voyage wasn't all that bad, now that I look back upon it. And looking back at this summer of fragile exile, I realize that, when I was not terrified, it was one of the happiest summers of my life. I was returning home to someone I had missed—my self.

AUTUMN

31

In western Maine, autumn begins when the last summer vacationers pack up their cars with fishing rods and damp bathing suits and a curtain of silence drops across the lake. It is the same every year, as comforting as porridge. Gone are the speedboats and jet-skis. Gone are the voices of strangers from canoes and docks. The loons return to our end of the lake and moan contentedly in the morning fog that hovers a few feet above the water. One day we watched three mallards paddling in formation at sunset, leaving golden jet streams behind their silhouettes in water as still as the ice it would soon become.

With the baby-sitters having returned to their own lives and Jack in Cambridge for his four-day workweek, I was alone with my alarm watch, knowing that in one press of the button an ambulance would come to save me. Silence filled the house and I wandered it aimlessly—confused, terrified, and delighted by my privacy and independence. It was the feeling I remembered from my first baby-sitting jobs: the parents would twirl out, leaving a hint of perfume and wool in the vestibule, and I would turn to their children with anxiety and excitement: So, what shall we do?

I reached for my summer schedule and clung to it, building my day around exercise and dutifully marching up and down our dirt driveway for the prescribed twenty minutes. Sometimes neighbors would take me walking on the main road in the warm sun under reddening sugar maples, a real treat.

Always in the back of my mind was the possibility of the box going off. If I left my alarm watch by the tub, I panicked and tried to walk calmly through the house to retrieve it, praying to the gods that this would not be the moment when the arrhythmia came back, wondering whether there would be enough time to press it as I dropped to the floor, ready for the hit. I found myself walking around always with a hand on something to steady me, a wall, a table, the banister. I moved quickly through open spaces and past sharp edges. I evaluated every surface underfoot for how well it would support or cushion me the next time I felt the jet revving up in my chest.

In her essay *On Being Ill*, Virginia Woolf wrote: "It is only the recumbent who knows what, after all, Nature is at no pains to conceal—that she in the end will conquer." Preparing for bed felt like a face-off with nature, the increasingly dark fall nights a time of reckoning for me. Lying very still, I would scan my body for signs of anything amiss. Had my heart always been this noisy? Had I always been able to watch it pulse beneath my breast? Was that thump an arrhythmia? Did the box repace it? Was my heart racing? Should I prepare for a hit? One morning I woke up on my back with my left arm behind my head as though I'd been enjoying the constellations. Thinking I had pulled the leads out of the ICD, I panicked and called my electrophysiologist. Jeremy assured me that the leads would only come out if I went back to work hurling garbage pails, as one of his patients had done.

As the house grew still, creaking occasionally from pressure changes, my longing for Jack's solid, life-affirming body became unbearable. It took real discipline to steady myself to face the darkness alone. I willed sleep to come fast, but my mind continued to explode with lit images. I was lucky: I never had nightmarish flashbacks from the operation as some patients do. I simply ricocheted from thought to incoherent thought.

Several times a night I woke to plan and carry out expeditions to the bathroom—first sitting at the edge of the bed (*Where am I?*), then slowly rising, pause, walking to the bedpost, pause, making my way across the carpet, passing through the door into the hall, holding onto the wall. It seemed to take an eternity and I always worried that I might not make it in time.

Illness is like a driving rain that forces you to stay indoors. On good nights I could calm myself by drawing on my yoga training to focus on my breath. In. Out. In. Out. So long as I could ignore the context, conscious breathing was an experience to be savored. Alone in our bed with only the sound of my own inhalations and exhalations, I was better able to return to the slowed-down place that had claimed me when I felt my chest tighten on May 12. More attuned to both body and soul than I'd ever been, I held on to this focus lest life and truth elude me. I began to understand the artistic temperament born of traveling into one's interior alone, the satisfaction and confidence it brings, the arrogance.

Jack was a wreck apart from me. He phoned at least ten times a day and called the local hospital if I didn't answer. We began long talks about how he had to begin to trust that all the protocols between our country hospital and MGH were in place. I reminded him that he would be the first person anyone would call if something went wrong, that my alarm watch could protect me better than he could because pros would be there in an instant, and that my Medic Alert bracelet was on my wrist forever. He stopped calling the hospital but would berate me for not answering the phone fast enough; I took to carrying it around in my apron pocket. Adding the phone to my portable arsenal was the least I could do to avoid causing Jack even a second of anxiety. I knew how important the sound of a voice was to restoring life.

Perri came over for a pajama party at least once a week after she had closed up the bookstore and arranged meals for her cats. It was comforting to have her spend the night—even though I knew full well that, in her eccentric Englishness, she would be a dithering disaster in a crisis and I would probably have to save *her*. It was worth the risk. She made me laugh. She brought me books. She let me feed her with no protests of "Stop. This is too much for you."

I spent all week thinking of the special meal I would have waiting for Jack when he zoomed down the driveway on Thursday afternoon—usually comfort food like meatloaf, which I never told him was made with organic ground turkey and buffalo meat from a farm nearby. I would leave our repast in the kitchen and wait for him on the porch like an excited first-grader watching for the bus to take her on a field trip. At the first crunch of gravel I was on my feet, beaming ecstatically. I'd watch Jack drive across the causeway much too fast, bumping high into the air on the frost heaves that one of Olga's

grandsons would soon bulldoze smooth in preparation for the coming winter.

I lift the top of the flour bin and shovel some into the big tan bowl
where a bubbling puddle of yeast is waiting. Bread baking is always
good for body and soul, and the crisp, clear air of late September has
made me yearn for a warm oven and the singular smell of freshly
baked bread. So here I am, delightedly up to my elbows in flour. I
work more and more in until it is too stiff to stir. Flipping the bowl
over is difficult, but I do it; the dough lands with a plop and a puff
of white. Joni Mitchell is playing on the stereo and Jack is coming
home tonight.

Slowly, tentatively, I begin to knead—paying attention to the place
where my arms meet my torso, observing my chest muscles and waiting for them to respond. My hands are deep in dough, but I am feeling
my body. The soft pile yields to my fingers and a rhythm begins to take
over as I push and pull gently, far less vigorously than in the old days.

My chest aches a little from the effort. It aches like it did last Sunday, when for the first time Jack rested on me again and I felt as vulnerable as I did at the first twisting of my chest when I had my MI. He held
most of his weight on his arms as we locked eyes in case this might be
our last view of each other, making love in the morning, the hour of
lovers who stay. It was neither a deliberate decision nor a reflex, but
a sudden, daring jump into a cold, bottomless quarry pool holding
hands. I can't say I felt my old fire-in-the-belly desire; the drugs were
suppressing that. I wept for not having died again.

Afterward, Jack's eyes were panicked and he tried to pull away
quickly to avoid putting any pressure on my breastbone. But I liked
him where he was. In illness, we were experiencing the skeleton of
love, the true bones of desire. I liked the ache.

Sex slowly, shyly returned to our life. We weathered its diminishment because it had always been the frosting on the cake. From our
first date—when we hadn't noticed the chairs being piled noisily on
tables all around us or the floor being washed by the late-night crew—
we began a conversation that we've never broken. After years of moon-
ing over some loser or a nice man who simply wasn't my destiny, I

now know that true love is when you are far more free and individual together than you ever would be apart. We flourish with no other company than each other, like children who happily whoop it up with their imaginary friends. Yet we know that we glow and attract people when they come near. We are a roaring hearth. I feel it in the heat of our sleep. A toe touching an ankle is electric.

32

IT IS MY FIRST REHAB CLASS at Maine Medical Center's Turning Point program. This will be my life three days a week for two months. Our housekeeper, Lil, has accepted the job of driving me the hour into Portland and back, and I am glad for my friend's comfort on the way to meet my new peer group, other cardiac patients. The tables are arranged in a horseshoe and my classmates all seem to be over sixty, except one wiry fellow about my age who confesses to eating six Big Macs for lunch regularly. There are several women, and I am surprised to find them here.

They revolt me.

What in the world am I doing with these sick people? I am not like them.

My nurse caseworker has kindly excused me from several of the classes—Shopping for Healthy Foods, Smoke and Smoking as a Risk Factor, and Meatless Meals.

Good. Because I could give the cooking class. I am not one of them. I am not.

We go around the room telling why we are there and what happened to us. Angioplasty, angina, stent (a small bridge placed in the artery to prevent it from collapsing), heart attack, scheduled open-heart surgery, single, double, triple bypass—terms that mean something to me now. Each of my classmates has a tale, most of them a singular experience with one of these classic cardiac "events."

I am last and rattle off my story like machine-gun fire. I went through all their ailments in one month. Behold the human wreck, left with cardiomyopathy and ventricular tachycardia.

There. Take that. See if you can top it. I smile sweetly. Aggressively. There is silence.

It felt good to get it out without crying, to say it all in one breath. My machine-gun report was exactly what it had been like: a high-speed rush of hellish, incomprehensible events. Telling strangers was an unexpected release, exposing a bitterness that I could never have expressed with people I knew.

In rehab I learned that heart disease is the number-one killer of American women. Wow. I had thought that heart attacks happen to women only in a vague, distant sense, probably when "they" are very, very old. A lot of women still believe this. Like them, I had thought that breast cancer would be my stalker. Wrong. Nearly dead wrong. As we now know, cardiovascular disease claims more women's lives than all cancers combined.

The now famous Framingham, Massachusetts study, which followed the health histories of generations of families, identified predictive factors for developing cardiovascular disease. Today these risk factors have been updated to include high blood pressure, high cholesterol, diabetes and pre-diabetes, smoking, an unhealthy diet, a sedentary lifestyle, excess weight, family history, age, race (African Americans, Mexican Americans, and Native Americans have a higher risk than Caucasians), and gender (women with a history of pre-eclampsia during pregnancy are prone and post-menopausal women are more prone than men).

When I had my MI in 1997, the list of predictive factors did not include stress. Today, some lists include uncontrolled stress (or anger), others do not. Stress is still regarded with some skepticism, at best a *trigger* if one or more of the other risk factors are present. So, since technically I had possessed none of the classic predictive factors, *Why me, indeed?*

It has been speculated that exhaustion can be a symptom of underlying heart disease, that clots may form more easily in people who are exhausted—and clots can cause dissections. But my vascular system was clean and I was not prone to clotting. Besides, Marc Semigran said there was no evidence that sturdy coronary arteries shred just because you are tired and strung out. I simply had to find some way to make peace with no explanation, with my heart attack as a freak event. Even so, the stress notion was like a mosquito in my ear at night as I tried to sleep.

My rehab training devoted an entire class to stress. There I learned that when we perceive danger—for example, a stranger following too closely on a dark and lonely street or a rumor circulating that the plant where we work is closing—a rapid-response system of physiological changes takes place within the body to enhance our ability to respond. This Stress Response is a survival trait we share with other mammals for those instances when, say, we are being chased by a lion. My classmates and I were learning how to counter it with the Relaxation Response, wonderfully deployed by simply breathing gently.

In 2013 I found a description in *Harvard Health Publications* of the Stress Response process as animated as those great biology cartoons we used to watch in grammar school. You know the ones, in which droplets of blood with smiley faces race through the vascular system as if they are riding a roller coaster. It all begins in the brain, the author(s) of "Understanding the Stress Response" explain—specifically in the amygdala, the area of the brain largely responsible for processing emotion.

A lion is charging!

Instantaneously, the amygdala sends a distress signal to the hypothalamus, "the command center." The hypothalamus communicates with the rest of the body through the autonomic nervous system. It has two messaging services to choose from in managing stress: the sympathetic nervous system (which functions as the gas pedal in a car) and the parasympathetic nervous system (the brake). Distress activates the sympathetic nervous system, which in turn signals the adrenal glands to pump more of the hormone epinephrine (also known as adrenaline) into the blood stream.

As epinephrine circulates, "the heart beats faster than normal, pushing blood to the muscles, heart, and other vital organs. Pulse rate and blood pressure go up. The person undergoing these changes also starts to breathe more rapidly. Small airways in the lungs open wide. This way the lungs can take in as much oxygen as possible with each breath. Extra oxygen is sent to the brain, increasing alertness. Sight, hearing, and other senses become sharper. Meanwhile, epinephrine triggers the release of blood sugar (glucose) and fats from temporary storage sites in the body. These nutrients flood into the bloodstream, supplying energy to all parts of the body."

What a magnificent readiness system! The Stress Response is why we can dodge an oncoming car or pull a child from a burning house before we even know we are moving. But this instantaneous cascade of responses is intended for extreme survival circumstances, not for a general lifestyle. To sustain a bodily state of high alert, the hypothalamus commands the sympathetic nervous system to press down harder on the gas pedal, releasing from the adrenal glands increased amounts of the "stress" hormone cortisol to keep the body revved up. When the threat passes, cortisol levels are supposed to fall and the parasympathetic nervous system is supposed to put the brakes on and restore the body to normal operations.

But what if we like the feeling of being on high alert? What if we gradually become accustomed to it, because of a lifestyle that keeps accelerating? What if we have no choice but to charge into battle or endure a forced march? Stress simply takes its toll—on our whole person.

Physician visionaries like Larry Dossey, Dean Ornish, Andrew Weil, and Herbert Benson were long considered the fringe of allopathic medicine with their insistence that what went on in our minds affected what went on in our bodies and vice versa. Today with mounting evidence that these visionaries and others were right, every major hospital is trying to find ways to incorporate lifestyle management and complementary care into preventing, treating, and helping patients to recover from all manner of disease and disability.

In 2014 Geoffrey H. Tofler, M.D. wrote a compelling article on the "Psychosocial Factors in Acute Myocardial Infarction" (*UpToDate*). He argues that the impact of stress should no longer be viewed with skepticism—listing study after study supporting a "causal link" between emotional upset/crisis or chronic stress and the incidence of MI. The examples are compelling, especially the results from one study: "There was a statistically significant 49 percent increase in patients admitted with MI through 16 emergency departments within a 50-mile radius of the World Trade Center in the 60 days after September 11, 2001, compared with the 60 days beforehand." It appears that the experience of disaster literally can break our hearts, though Dr. Tofler cautions that "the mechanism" as to how this exactly happens "is uncertain."

Back in 1997 as I shakily went through the paces of my rehab program based on Dr. Herbert Benson's Mind/Body connection, it was becoming abundantly clear to me that leaving the adrenal tap open to flow with stress hormones cannot help but have a corrosive effect on the body as well as the mind. In my controlled study of one, I could feel the difference in my own body after one summer of peace. It was plain to me that a chronic state of "fight or flight" is simply not good for anyone's health.

But, surely I had been under no more stress than anyone leading an overloaded, productive work life in Boston! Had my life really been more alienating than any frequent flyer's, wheeling a bag through stale, glaring, beeping airports? More than any woman with a complex family with complex issues?

Marc once again assured me that sturdy coronary arteries do not shred just because we have a plane to catch.

Besides, I rationalized to myself, stress is a single mother unable to give her kids a secure life, not a thriving professional who can pay the bills, right? Stress is Africans struggling with the outbreak of a deadly virus without medical assistance, or refugees fleeing genocide, or the lives of my doctors who never sleep. Stress could not possibly be coming home to a marriage that is a deep and delightful oasis.

Yet the rehab program on stress rang all kinds of bells that clanged in my head. When I learned about the relationship between stress and the immune system, I could no longer ignore the constant colds leading up to my heart attack. Surely these were warnings that something was terribly wrong, no matter what had actually caused my LAD to dissect.

I had taken everything to heart! Yes, that was it. Even that expression was a warning in hindsight. Yet it was also true that my tendency to engage deeply also made me a compassionate friend, a reliable worker, a principled citizen. There is such a thing as good stress, isn't there?

Isn't there?

In her book *Heart: A Personal Journey Through Its Myths and Meanings*, Gail Godwin offers an insight into what exactly constitutes a healthy pace as we go about our daily rounds. She writes, "The Italians have a musical notation not found in any other language: *tempo giusto*, 'the right tempo.' It means a steady, normal beat, between 66 and 76 on the metronome. *Tempo giusto* is the appropriate beat of the human heart."

As I was learning in rehab, the beat of a healthy heart at rest and at peace is even slower, about 60 beats per minute. I began to pay attention to any beat: drums, footsteps, a knock at the door, and I discovered something magical. We can hear *tempo giusto* in the tick of the second hand as it makes its way around the clock and in the rhythm of a bride's step as she walks down the aisle to her beloved. The beat of a healthy human heart is the beat we have chosen to accompany both time and love, our most precious commodities.

One day a friend noisily blasted through our front door with enough energy to fling me out of the *tempo giusto* I was trying to cultivate. Using a new trick that I had learned during Mind/Body training, we did an experiment. I measured her heart rate and found it to be more than one hundred beats a minute. Then she kindly, indulgently, closed her eyes and was quiet for just a few minutes. Her heart rate returned to *tempo giusto*! What's more, she felt much better, calmer and more capable of handling her troubles. But how many of us buzz chronically, mercilessly racing our hearts and destroying our health, not to mention our enjoyment of time and love?

After class, I cornered one of my rehab instructors, because she had perfectly described my life pre-heart attack. Maybe she had the answer! Did she think that stress had done me in?

Rather than answer my question, she gazed at me serenely, without judgment, and I thought, *I want that. I want to learn how she does that.*

Poison is not a good substance to keep inside you, and the body usually expels it one way or another. Emotional poison needs a little help toward the exit, too. When Marc discharged me from the hospital, he had suggested that I might find a little therapy useful in my adjustment. MGH referred me to a Portland psychiatrist and I dumped my grief in Karen's office for eight weeks every Friday following rehab.

From the very first session, the click of her door closing was like a slap between the shoulder blades. I began to cry immediately, bitterly, with Karen as my only witness, flooding her serene room with the violent waters that were drowning me inside. Finally, after a couple of sessions, we could talk. Week after week, I laid regrets, questions, terror, and anger on the table for us to examine, while the tears kept spilling out. I was shocked at the depth of the feelings my broken heart had unleashed. Unfinished business rises like heat in any crisis, especially a life-threatening medical crisis, because when the core of life itself is vulnerable, the patient can't help but question its meaning, a much larger topic than the body.

I've always cried spontaneously in the presence of truth, whether truth presents itself in the form of beautiful music, the insightful comment of a friend, or a moving book. The truth that rose from my time with Karen was simple and profound: at the core of my sadness and anger was not the loss of my own good health, but another, earlier loss. Dylan Thomas wrote, "After the first death there is no other." My mother's death was the first death, and my new tears were seemingly unstoppable because they were mixed with the old to create a current as strong as the meeting of two rivers. My heart attack had given me permission, finally, to fall apart, something I should have done years earlier.

There we were, all six of us, in the vestibule of St. Mary's church, ages thirteen to three. It was overflowing—like the funeral of President Kennedy that we had seen on TV. But Mum had watched that funeral with us and we had all cried together. Now she was the one in the polished coffin. We saw her sleeping in there at the wake, wearing Robbie's macaroni pin on her favorite teal dress that showed off her green eyes, if only she would open them.

We rode to her funeral in a black limousine like the Kennedys. The chauffeur was wearing a black uniform and helped me step from the backseat as big as a bathroom. I adjusted my black mantilla and felt glamorous, unsure of my age. Blurred faces crowded the sidewalk. I wondered whether Johnny was the altar boy that day. I hoped not, in case I cried. That would be embarrassing.

Before the funeral procession began, Dad pulled us into a huddle and told each and every one of us not to cry, not to let him down. *Anything for you, Dad*—our desperately sad Dad, sole line of defense against dreaded nannies with warts, dark orphanages, and separation among the relatives. *Which aunt would I choose to live with? Would I have a choice? Where would I sleep?* I imagined the crowded houses of my cousins. There was no place to go but the orphanage. *Anything for you, Dad*—our protector who had cried in front of us for the first time, his face contorted as though he'd eaten something bad and wanted to vomit.

Thus began an innocent conspiracy to suppress grief in our family, to put on a brave face for the world. As the eldest, I led the charge, layering on more and more responsibility, exploding in anger, lying with laughter, burying my spirit with my mother while working harder and harder to replace her and wondering why it was never enough. None of us cried openly for years except for Leesa, the teariest child I have ever known. She saw us walking around with gold stars on our frozen foreheads while she soaked her pillow with secret tears of grief. And she cried in front of people, too. How embarrassing. All it took was a kind glance, a question harmlessly directed her way.

I have always believed that each and every one of us is responsible for doing her own emotional homework, for doing the best we can with our gifts and constraints. The process of facing down our ghosts is our small, attainable contribution to a kinetic process that holds the potential for healing the world. And why not? After all, the opposite is true: history has proven that people who are unwilling to catch and release their individual sadnesses, disappointments, and hidden motivations have compensated by wreaking havoc on the world. Good and evil lies within each of us, and every day we choose which potential to fulfill.

So, bolstered with a deeper understanding of the impact of "the first death," my mother's, and invited to look deeper by the realization that I had lived at the same age that she had died, I returned to my cloister of physical weakness more open than ever to what I might find there.

33

It is a brilliant September afternoon and Jack has just tucked me into the hammock for a snooze. Underneath me is a matted plaid blanket that I stole from the school where I taught in Switzerland because it comforted me there and I had never stolen anything before. Over me is a soft mohair throw the color of sunlight on brick woven by my friend Ann. The sun is warm and I feel a little cool air on the inch of bare skin between my socks and jeans. The sky rains golden needles with each gentle sway of the white pines overhead. Soon they will cover the paths through the huckleberry bushes, muting sound. Then they'll turn russet and smell of sweet decay. I feel my life curling around the seasons, feel myself beginning to trust that the next one will follow.

And then I see it.

My husband has planted a second apple sapling in the sour soil of our shade-covered, windswept pine grove—a hellish environment for any fruit-bearing tree, even the sturdy New England apple. A few years ago he installed the first one, lovingly digging a hole just so and filling it with compost to give it the best start possible. Today it is barely five feet tall and scrawny, bent from constant pummeling by the Canadian winds. Occasionally the tree boasts tiny leaves. It never blooms.

Now it has a mate. We read recently that apple trees need old-fashioned sex, that they will bloom only if both male and female are present. I know without examining it (how would I examine it anyway?) that this is the chosen life-companion for Tree Number One, a symbolic planting. Jack has placed them two feet away from each other: snuggling distance for people, strangling distance for trees. And he has planted in autumn, giving the lover little hope of settling in before winter freezes its roots to death. But like me, that tree just might have a chance. Jack's will is a force to be reckoned with when he sets his heart on something.

That's another one: "sets his heart on something."

In my search for the meaning of my MI, I have become sensitive to the manifold uses of the word "heart," listing expressions and phrases and staring at them like ancient runes. For example, I have discovered that heart and earth are permutations of each other. In its Old English derivation, *heorte* referred to the center of all vital functions—not just a muscle, but the seat of affection, desires, and thoughts, the center of love, the core of spirit and manifestation of the divine. Its meaning is the same in most languages. I have also learned that the French use *coeur*, heart, figuratively the same way that we do—to be openhearted, to take heart, to memorize by heart. If you look at the etymology of the word *coeur*, you can also see that it is related to the word "courage." Richard the Lionhearted. (Come to think of it, the many uses of "heart" may be the only subject on which the French and English can agree.)

A friend once told me, "You live from the heart." She was somewhat sad in her observation, which puzzled me at the time. Now that I had been punched in the chest, I had all the time in the world to consider what she meant.

Today is Lil's day to work at the nursing home, so Perri has volunteered to drive me to rehab, since she has a day off from the bookstore. Driving along in my old red car the size of a skate, we learn more about each other. For example, I discover that Perri cannot do two things at the same time; the more animatedly she talks, the slower she drives. I know we are in trouble when she begins to gesture with both hands. As a truck with a large man and black dog speeds by us, I look at the speedometer—we are driving 20 mph in a 50 mph zone. Then I look in the rearview mirror and see the cars lined up behind us. My car still has Massachusetts plates and I just know we are adding to Maine's antipathy toward flatlanders' driving. I slouch down a little in the front seat to strategize. We are going to be late for the nine o'clock class.

She looks at the clock on my dashboard. "It can't be eight-thirty already!"

We are going to be late. "Perri, drive just a little faster."

And she does, at least until we get talking again. I pepper our lively conversation with reminders about where to turn, when to pass, stop, and go, and which lane to drive in. I even point out a good place for a haircut.

"I know. I told you about it, Deborah."

It's quarter to nine, and we are still a half hour away. She looks at her own watch.

"Deborah, could your clock be fast? Mine shows only eight-thirty."

And then I remember. To prevent tardiness in the land of the healthy, I set all our clocks to different times—except Jack's watch and the digital clock in his car, which he declared off limits. Perri has caught me out; my car clock was set fifteen minutes ahead.

In the parking lot, giggling, we fumble for a pen and use the tip to reset the clock to the exact time. For the first time in years I am conscious of living in the moment, liberated like Gracie the parrot above the fields on Martha's Vineyard. I have taken back time.

It is not until a year later, over a bottle of wine, that Perri—who drives to Portland at least weekly—admits to biting her tongue as I bossed her around. She figured I was still adjusting, she says.

Like the cloistered, I spent my time in contemplation and wore the same clothes every day. I considered the coincidences that had led me to this moment in time, beginning with my mother's death at forty-four, the same age I was when I had my heart attack. Then there was Jack's birthday, September 22, the very day my mother had died. And I thought about our months of agonizing about whether to conceive a child or not. It was a tough enough question, considering our ages and the fact that we already had Jack's five kids, but when Jack began to have nightmares of my dying in childbirth, I decided this was one dream I could give up. I had married him for love, not for children. Besides, grandchildren were already here. It turns out that Jack's anxiety was well founded. Because I was born with a defective coronary artery, I most likely would have died in childbirth.

I considered the string of circumstances that led me to diagnose myself and get swift cardiac care, stemming from our friend Tom's absence at our annual February climb of Mount Washington. His wife had rushed him to the hospital with chest discomfort, which turned out to be a muscle pull from skiing like a demon the day before. This prompted me to pay attention to a *Fortune* article, on heart attacks that I picked up on an airplane a few weeks later. I had cut the article out and sent it to Tom, memorizing the symptoms in case Jack ever had them.

For the month before my MI, we had both been in Europe on business, and then on vacation. It had not happened in a lonely Italian vineyard or on the plane back. Either scenario would have meant certain death. At the time of my heart attack, I was supposed to be on a plane to Detroit, but just a few days before my meeting had been changed to a phone conference. My lower back had been aching and I almost went to the chiropractor instead of to yoga class. The class had only two people in it; usually there were at least eight. I had the teacher's full attention, and her training told her never to ignore the body. I was minutes from Mount Auburn Hospital. Those minutes saved my life because my MI reached its devastating climax in the emergency room.

There were still more coincidences. When Jack moved to Boston to marry me, a fledgling company called Genzyme hired him. At the time he knew nothing about biotechnology, and joked that he thought DNA was a rock group. His colleagues would later help assemble a stellar team of doctors for me at MGH. Adding profoundly to the eeriness of all these coincidences, I came out of anesthesia on May 20, our eighth wedding anniversary. And Jack unwittingly moved me to Maine to begin my new life on June 27, my forty-fifth birthday.

I had always believed that Jack was my mother's gift to me. Every September 22, I looked to the heavens and thanked her as I filled his birthday cake with cinnamon-and-sugar-coated apples. But with the full lineup of coincidences, my search for *why* turned metaphysical. Did the heart attack occur to eject me from a business life at odds with my soul? Did the weight of the world have to be wrenched from me before I could let go? Was the whole horrible adventure a gift from my dead mother to break the spell of grief and silence that had plagued our family for thirty-two years?

As a child, I had been told that "everything happens for a reason" and it is not for us to ask why. I can hear my two generations of aunts saying this solemnly—as though they knew why my pet salamander lay shriveled in its box, and I was simply too young to understand. I always hated the passivity of that explanation. At the time, of course, I had no idea of its roots in a fatalism shared by many faiths that an all-knowing god has a grand plan for each of us. Now despite being agnostic (or perhaps because of it), I could not ignore the collection of coincidences that had somehow conspired to save my life, as though things really did happen for a reason.

Were my observations of serendipity—or synchronicity, as intuitive healer Caroline Myss would say—a product of my Catholic upbringing, a secret yearning for a god who takes care of things for us? Or were they the product of personality, my habit of turning lemons into lemonade and trying to find something positive about every mess? Or, is there some underlying order to the universe, divine or otherwise, that determines how all things turn out?

Jack once asked this question of renowned biologist and Pulitzer Prize winner Edward O. Wilson (following a lecture he gave at Harvard University with his old intellectual and funding rival James D. Watson, who with Francis Crick received a 1962 Nobel Peace Prize for describing the double helix structure of DNA).

Dr. Wilson's answer: "Who knows, Jack? What do you think?"

Amen. I prefer the questions. They invite us to pay attention. As I reflected, and read, and incorporated more of my cardiac rehab lessons into my life, I noticed that my mind was learning to apply from yoga practice what my body had already demonstrated by saving my life: the power of paying attention. And the more I paid attention, the more I discovered that there is meaning and connection everywhere, if we bother to look.

34

JULIANA, MARK, HILLERY, AND GEORGE arrived in early October for the opening day of the Fryeburg Fair, the longest-running agricultural fair in the United States, rumored to be where Fern showed Wilbur in E.B. White's *Charlotte's Web*.

Going to the fair was my idea. Our guests were not sure whether I had the stamina for it, but I insisted. It just wasn't autumn without a day at the fair. My favorite event is the pig scramble, where small and large children chase after squealing baby pigs. The rules are simple: if you catch one, you take it home. There is nothing that makes me laugh as hard as watching those kids fling their tiny, tough bodies into the air after a panicked baby pig that does not yet realize it will be loved as much as Fern loved Wilbur.

We parked on the back road and began our walk toward the east fair gate. Our route took us through the parking lot of RVs and trailers that were the homes of people running the Ferris wheel and selling cotton candy, people who had brought animals to show, the man who sold chopping knives with the zeal of a revival preacher, women whose gleaming jars of summer's bounty would be judged sternly. It was a friendly, honky-tonk village with all the comforts of home—folding chairs and awnings, real mums and plastic daisies. Some had toted motorcycles on the back of their RVs for quick trips to the grocery store.

I was filled with excitement but tried to pace myself. I hadn't noticed how long this walk was before. Neither had Jack. Halfway through the lot, we realized our mistake: I needed to save my energy for walking around the fair, not getting to it. Just then, miraculously, we spotted a golf cart with a white-haired lady dressed in pink perched in the backseat, clutching her bag like the Queen Mother. *Handicapped access!* Jack hailed it. The driver looked puzzled at a slim young woman climbing up to ride shotgun but didn't ask questions.

I didn't care what anyone thought; I was delighted. *Tallyho driver! We're going to the fair.*

As we entered, children were lining up with their steers for the parade past the viewing stands. The steers jostled and tossed their heads from the weight of their fancy yokes, occasionally reminded to behave by the swat of a willow branch. The kids were proud, serious. Hillery kissed the nose of nearly every animal, smitten.

We bought a huge pile of onion rings and I ate one whole, crusty, greasy ring. We went carefully through the arts and crafts tent for treasures. For Christmas, I bought a cute knit hat with ear flaps for Jack's grandson Cotter, which he would later declare to be a very cool snowboarding hat. I bought a cedar-needle-filled pillow for Jack's mother and Johnson jackets, those ubiquitous black-and-red New England plaid wool shirt-jackets, for Mary Kate's brood.

And then Jack looked long and hard into my eyes. After only an hour and a half I was unraveling quickly. The crowds felt suddenly oppressive. I grew pale and shaky. Sleep was coming on as fast as a squall.

"We have to get her out of here. Now," Jack said to Juliana, reading me like the sky.

Juliana went to find the others while I stumbled to the nearest gate on Jack's arm. I was amazed and ashamed at the rapidity of my descent. It had been a telling debut: ordinary events were no longer ordinary for me. I had stayed too long at the fair. *That's okay. Now I know.*

The ticket taker had his back to us, focused on people arriving. Behind him was a stool. I lunged for it and Jack helped settle me in. Then we asked permission. No, the man didn't mind a bit. With Jack gone to fetch the car, the man took it upon himself to keep up a steady stream of chatter with his back to me, amiably keeping me company while he took tickets and stamped hands. He didn't notice that I was asleep, leaning on my basket of presents.

That week we called Marc to ask his opinion about a "handicapped" placard for our car. He agreed it was a wise idea—no point in wasting precious energy simply getting to a destination. We submitted the required papers and the state responded quickly, sending a placard we could hang on the rearview mirror of either of our two cars. We had a moment of depression about it—just until the next time we went to MGH and slipped into a handicapped parking space. After another grueling day at the hospital showing off how fine I was in the face of tests that said otherwise, the car parked right next to the elevator on the fourth floor of the garage was a gift.

Steven, who was about to move to Cambridge, where parking was scarce, suggested that we make laminated copies of the placard and give it to all our friends for Christmas.

35

IT IS THE LAST DAY OF REHAB CLASSES. Lil and I are laughing as the elevator doors open and we separate—Lil to read her Bible in the waiting room and I to join my buddies in the rehab gym. It didn't take me long to love these nice people after my horrified first day. I will miss them. I've even gotten to know some spouses who join the classes, encouraged by Turning Point to make what is often a family lifestyle change. Like Teeno and Jean. They make me think of Jack Sprat, who ate no fat, and his wife, who ate no lean. A strong, wiry man, Teeno was collecting fiddleheads deep in the woods when he had his heart attack and he walked all the way back to the house. Jean is so large that she can barely move, swollen with every kind of ailment from diabetes to hypertension to chronic angina. She had her own turn in the hospital a few years back but didn't go to rehab. Teeno's enrollment encouraged her to join, too. But she isn't here today. *Odd, the last class . . .*

One day, when he was not working, Jack went to class with me. I was proud to show him off and glad to have a second pair of ears in the session on medications, which continue to baffle me. But when the instructor began to talk, Jack began to giggle. Then he tickled me and kneaded my thigh suggestively. I pounded his knee under the table, yet he persisted in acting like the class clown. I could not believe it. Not only had I missed precious explanations of the chemistry experiment I had become, but I couldn't count on my rock. I was alone after all. And mad. I hissed into his ear that I wanted him to leave and he instantly woke up, eyes filled with remorse. It had been a classic stress reaction. I determined then and there that I would find him counseling. Enough of this strong-man bullshit.

But that troubling incident is far from my mind today as I climb onto the treadmill. The hardest thing is turning it on. Lisa, our nurse-trainer, helps me and I begin to walk, bouncing a little on the rubber. I turn up the speed and increase the grade. My breathing is a little more labored now. I stay at that level until it feels good, then pick up the speed some more.

"Almost on target, Deborah," says Lisa, reading the central machine that monitors our heart rates as we work out. The target heart rate for exercise is calculated at 60 to 75 percent of a person's maximum heart rate. To determine what that is, they measure one's heart rate at rest and then at maximum exertion during a treadmill stress test supervised by a physician. Then the data is plugged in to something called the Karvonene Formula to yield a range.

"Good, now you're in your target range."

I keep moving at that pace, memorizing the feeling for next week, when I will be on my own again. Our eight weeks of classes have been important in training our bodies to know instinctively when we are at the right pace. In my case, I have to be careful not to exceed it. Unlike my compatriots, I know what it is to feel good, and my body naturally seeks the rush of intensive aerobic activity now forbidden to me.

To help keep me in my target range when I do my walks at home, I've bought an athlete's heart monitor, which straps around my chest. Once set, the watch that comes with it beeps if you go below or above your target rate. I asked the saleswoman at the bike shop where I bought it to set it to 94 to 98 beats per minute and she thought I was joking. "But that's barely moving! I'm not sure this system goes that low." It was depressing to feel judged by a stranger.

"What's your RPE, Deborah?" Lisa shouts to me above the whirring of her marathoners.

"Four." Four means "somewhat hard" and indicates a good workout. Without a professional guiding me, I'd be afraid to push myself like this.

RPE, or Rate of Perceived Exertion on the Borg scale of one to ten, is a person's subjective assessment of how hard he or she is working, incorporating both exertion and fatigue. It can take the place of taking the pulse. An RPE of greater than five or the inability to have a light conversation while exercising usually indicates overexertion. Walking daily at a clip for thirty minutes, within my range of 94 to 98 beats per minute, is my new prescription.

With the bypass, the box, my alarm watch, the phone in my apron pocket, and now my athlete's monitor, I have become the bionic woman. A new pair of sneakers used to be as high-tech as I got.

After fifteen minutes my fingers are still freezing, but soon they'll

be warm as the blood reaches my extremities. I feel the sweat starting as my feet rhythmically hit the treadmill. I was so proud of my
twenty-minute workouts on the driveway during the summer. Little
did I know that I was moving at a snail's pace. But the practice was
critical; it built me up to take full advantage of my training at Turning
Point. And look at me blaze now!

"Hey, show-off," my buddy Rodney yells from the next treadmill,
"trying to make the rest of us look like slugs?"

We all tease each other. Actually, I am amazed at how well my
classmates are moving, spurring me to do better. I *am* younger, after
all. We compete with each other without realizing it and it's good for
us. By the end of the workout I am high as a kite. We all are! Everyone
is smiling and laughing.

As I move into the circle we form for cool-down exercises and
meditation, I pass the chart with our individual data and sneak a peek.
Feeling at the top of my game, I cannot resist comparing myself to the
others on graduation day.

Suddenly I feel very still inside.

My numbers are worse than everyone's—worse than Jean's, and
we've just learned that she is absent because she's been hospitalized
again. I picture her heaving her way into the circle and I grip the back
of my chair. *So, I'm really sick. This is not going away.* My ejection fraction and target heart rate are even lower than Jean's, and she can barely
walk. Then I remember that this is old data from when I first left the
hospital. The tests in Boston in two weeks will surely show a difference. How else could I be doing this well? I shake off the fear and calm
myself with our last meditation practice. When we open our eyes we
smile woozily at one another.

In eight short weeks, my new friends have had to change their
diets completely, stop smoking, and include forty minutes of exercise
in their daily routine. It's a lot to keep track of—on top of medications,
stress management, and the other myriad adjustments, which are
overwhelming. Several must balance the work of rehabilitation with
jobs and family responsibilities. Some of them are alone, or do not
have supportive families. Some have been suffering from cardiovascular disease their whole lives, while I managed to make it to forty-four

without a hitch. I admire their courage, strength, and humor. They've helped me to see sparkles on the swamping waves.

As my gift to them, I've brought a brightly wrapped copy of *The Mediterranean Diet Cookbook* by my friend Nancy Harmon Jenkins, an expert on eating well and healthily. I've also brought slips of paper scribbled with my fellow graduates' names. I announce that we are holding a raffle and we fumble for someone's baseball cap. I have inscribed the cookbook, "You are not on a diet, you are on an extended tour of the Mediterranean." Bon voyage!

For the next couple of weeks, I thought about Jean, Teeno's wife, constantly. I called Turning Point a few times and learned that she was still in intensive care. We used to change into our exercise clothes together while exchanging pleasantries, medical tips, and complaints, nothing too intimate. Being in class for a life-threatening disease was our bond; we were both training for our lives. Before leaving for Boston, I called Turning Point to find out if she was out of intensive care yet so I could send flowers. She had just died. I was stunned. Rehab classes had been a return to school, and you never expect the girl in line next to you in gym to die. It means you are vulnerable, too.

36

I AM PLEASED TO RETURN TO MGH to show off my progress after these six months. Physically, I almost fit in with the visitors I see walking around. I'm a little skinny, and my shoulders still fold in like a fallen maple leaf, but I can pass. Part of me feels like I can handle anything; the other part is jittery. The numbers still rule and these tests are important.

First to the pulmonary lab. I contort my mouth to fit around a plastic harmonica, and Tatiana asks me to blow into it.

"That's nice," she says. Tatiana is from Russia and her accent is luscious. She is wearing a little black dress under her lab coat.

"Very good. Again. Blow, blow, blow, get all of it out." I remember doing this before. But I didn't walk into the lab then; I was wheeled in on a gurney. As I blow, blow, blow, I privately celebrate being an "ambulatory care" patient.

"Good. Very good."

"How good?"

"Your tests are much better than last time. In fact, you test almost like a normal, healthy person. Congratulations. Dr. Semigran will have these results in time for your appointment."

The heart and lungs work as a team in the thoracic cavity, pumping vital oxygen throughout the body. If my lungs are strong, it means that so far they are handling with aplomb the work that my heart can't do. All those weeks of blowing into my lung toy and walking have made a difference. I float out of the lab, lightly touching Jack's arm. I have become enchanted.

Next I visit the electrophysiology lab. From this day forward, my ICD will be tested annually. It is my big date with death. After putting me under general anesthesia, the electrophysiologist will race my heart to see first if the box correctly attempts to repace it. Then he'll race my heart so it pushes through the barrier into full ventricular fibrillation to find out whether the box fires to save my life.

Will I ever get used to this? I am coldly terrified, a lamb to slaughter.

In the waiting room, a woman in her late thirties is looking pale and tense.

"Are you all right?" I ask.

"I'm just a little nervous. Thanks for asking. My husband is being tested in there," she nods her head toward the lab door. "He has an atrial arrhythmia and they test him every now and again. I hate it. He's always cheerful about it. You'd think I was the one undergoing the test."

People live a long time with atrial fibrillation, an uneven and rapid heartbeat in the atrial chamber of the heart. It can be controlled with medication, though the heart's fluttering is unnerving, can cause fainting, and in the extreme can be life-threatening. In serious cases, like her husband's, patients are monitored. On the other hand, ventricular tachycardia, the condition I developed during surgery, has no ambiguity. It simply results in sudden cardiac death, unless you have an ICD.

To stall my own panic, I draw her out. She tells me that they have been married for ten years, have two small children, are deeply in love. That he can be macho about illness and pain. That she has to watch him like a hawk. That the doctors say he can live his whole life healthily with his condition. That he's never even had a heart attack, thank God.

He emerges—large and male and vibrant.

"See what 1 mean?" She turns to me as he enfolds her in his arms. "He's not even drowsy like he should be. Oh, I'm so sorry, I didn't even ask you why *you* are here." She looks at my silver-haired husband.

"Oh, just a little test." Jack replies, squeezing my hand. The couple walks out the door, wrapped around each other.

"You all right?" Jack peers at me and I don't have time to answer because a nurse is ushering me into the lab, leaving Jack to wait beside the piles of magazines.

I am shivering inside, and it's not just the flimsy johnny. I wonder if it shows as I greet my old EP buddies warmly. It shows. They turn up the heat and tuck blankets around my frigid toes. They attach an external defibrillator to my body and insert an IV in my arm. Then they begin to administer the general anesthesia that will knock me out. Jeremy is here now. Everything is much better with him beside me.

I suddenly need reassurance about the future. "Jeremy, you said that when I come back here in five years to have the battery changed, instead you may insert a whole new defibrillator the size of a quarter, right?"

He looks up from my chart. "They're working on it."

Wow. A couple of years before it was the size of a deck of cards and would have been inserted in my belly. By the time of my procedure, it was the size of a cigarette lighter. I got the right disease. It is my last thought before I go to sleep.

I awake from a beautiful, hallucinogenic dream with a smile on my face. Flowers. Fairies. Great drugs. There have been no arrhythmias and the box fired just fine. "It works!" they tell me cheerily. I am supposed to feel great about this. I do, I do, I do. See you next year! Next patient please. The happy, Technicolor dream is over and I feel gray.

After a rest and lunch, I am ready for the nuclear lab. The nuclear test is defining. It will tell us what my ejection fraction is, a number I've been working very hard to improve with my daily discipline of rest and exercise. The left ventricle, the part of my heart that is severely damaged, is the powerhouse of the heart and determines the EF. If the EF is going to rise at all after surgery, it will do so immediately and perhaps a little more in the first three months. In most cases, after three months it will stay put. It's been five months since my last test. I'll soon know if I still have half the heart of the average American.

I *know* that I have advanced from my measly 25 percent, but it would be nice to have scientific proof. If only Marc could see me on my speed-walks, he would know I am almost all better now.

The technician attempts to draw blood for a benchmark. He can't get a vein and sticks me a few times as I turn the color of rain. He is damp and doesn't look much better than me.

"I'm sorry, but you have to ask someone else to do this. I'm a 'hard stick.' It's not your fault," I say.

The words "hard stick" work instantly—like throwing around the occasional *bon* or *d'accord* on vacation in France. The technician returns with the man who saved him months before when I was wheeled in on a gurney and could not roll onto the test platform by myself. The pro succeeds on the first try, then injects me with the radioactive tracer fluid. Like the last time, he assures me it is a very tiny, safe dosage, but I think of Chernobyl. I return to the waiting room with Jack while the fluid makes its way through my body.

Then I am under the torpedo again, trying not to move for three ten-minute intervals, not even a nose twitch. I'm a pro this time, drawing on the meditation training from rehab classes. Before I know it, the test is done.

We go for a cup of tea to revive me. Then we make our weary way into the Bullfinch Building for a quick social visit with Torch. We wait and wait, needing his larger-than-life presence to reassure us that we are doing as well as we think we are. But Torch never shows; there are complications with some struggling soul on the operating table and Torch puts in another twenty-four-hour day. Just as well. I am so utterly drained that he would not be encouraged by how I look right now.

When we were here in September and saw him coming down the hall toward us, I broke into a run. He looked stricken. "Marc isn't allowing you to run, is he?" And then I remembered all my instructions, forgotten in a moment of pure joy. *No. No, he isn't.* No sudden bursts of happiness. No sprinting, not even toward my torch of light.

With difficulty, I make Jack take me back to the SICU (surgical intensive care unit). Jack does not want to go there again, ever. I prevail; it's another important exorcism. The elevator ejects us and he leads me down the hall past the big silver OR elevator where he kissed me goodbye. He shows me the SICU waiting room that became the family camp. I had imagined it large and soft, but it is a tiny, cold room with rigid chairs against the wall. Then Jack leads me along the corridor toward the main desk, past rooms with swollen lumps under blankets wired to machines. It is a quiet floor. We walk by my old room and I remember the feeling of it. I lose myself in the body lying there now. In another room, five or so people are working swiftly on one of the lumps.

At the main desk, an aide is writing a report and looks up. He smiles very slowly, staring at me.

"I know your eyes," he says. And I remember him. He came to lift me and was gentle.

A nurse scurries out when she sees strangers talking with the aide and asks if she can help us.

"You already have," I say. "I am Deborah Heffernan."

And Joanne is in my arms, tiny Joanne who is even tinier now that I am on my feet and holding her body in mine. *It's Joanne!* Other nurses and aides appear, grinning slowly with recognition, staring in disbelief. One cups my narrow, bony face in her hands and says, "But you're so *thin.*" And I am brought swiftly back to a time when I would not have recognized myself, grotesquely swollen into a ghoul. We all cry and Jack turns away, overcome. It was a good idea to come back. Good for Jack and me, good for my care-givers. They needed to see a success.

187

Drained, the two of us gravitate to the Ellison-8 waiting room to rest before the walk to Marc's office for my final appointment of the day. I do not want to arrive in a wheelchair. I want to sail in vigorous and proud with the spinnaker full and flags snapping. I curl into a ball and am asleep instantly.

"He stashes chocolates everywhere. We're forever finding them and taking them away. He's really tall, but he'll be big as a house if he's not careful," the technician chatters, solicitous of Marc, while she hooks me up to the EKG machine.

"Ever notice his white jackets? He can't button them and his arms stick out. We try to put aside the big ones and launder them ourselves so he doesn't look so silly. But he never even notices. Marc is just focused on his patients. He's a good man."

We smile knowingly at each other and I begin to think of ways to influence Marc's diet. He is forty-three and I need him to stay well for a long, long time. It's funny how doctors rarely practice what they preach. Marc asked me to drink only a couple of glasses of wine a week because my liver is being taxed by the drugs. And he binges on chocolate? Well, I enjoy a glass of red wine with dinner every night, justifying it with the latest studies promoting the cardiac benefits of cabernet sauvignon.

Marc walks in reading my chart. We weigh me. Back up to 128. That's good. But he warns me to stay under 130 for awhile. I look like a scrawny chicken, but if he likes me that way, so be it. He checks my ankles for swelling and listens to my chest and lungs. My blood pressure is nice and low. I am bursting with curiosity, ready to levitate the minute I hear the undoubtedly great result of the nuclear test.

"So, you had your EF test today," he says in his slightly singsong way, smiling much too nicely. "I have the results here. And you've gone up a bit—from 25 to 28."

"Great!" I am so ready for good news that I do not absorb what he has just said. I strain forward, a silly smile frozen on my face.

"Well, yes, we like to see the numbers go up," he continues carefully. "But this change is actually statistically insignificant, Deb. Each time we do the test, there will be some variation due to circumstances. We look for major changes. So . . ."

Jack is as still as I am. The room begins to blur.

So my EF is the same.

I see Jean heaving about in rehab, and her EF was better than mine. This can't be true: my EF hasn't budged since I left the hospital in a wheelchair? All my new tricks have made no difference.

"So I am going to die."

"No, no, no!" says Marc. "Many people lead long lives with ejection fractions like yours, with varying degrees of limitation."

He can see that I am struggling with the word "limitation." Being a scientist, he knows there is hope in technology, so he elaborates.

"And when your other organs begin to tire and rebel because of the extra work they are doing, we still have options. We can move on to a transplant."

A what?

I shoot Jack a look of betrayal. Have you known this all along? Jack shoots the accusing look back to Marc.

"I thought that when she had her double bypass we avoided the transplant. What are you saying, Marc?"

"That's true. The bypass avoided the transplant she needed *then*. But it was only a temporary measure to save her life in the immediate, Jack."

I don't recognize Jack. He has become Alice in Wonderland after eating the biscuit, bewildered and tiny.

Marc continues as delicately as possible. "We've said this all along, but I understand completely that the possibility receded for you with her progress, Jack. The transplant has always been an option. And I'm glad that it is. You have to look at it this way: there is hope."

I'm supposed to be happy that I can get a transplant? Do I kick up my heels with glee? Marc has lost his mind. Who is this "she" they are talking about?

I speak to him in a small furry voice from far away. "When will I need a heart transplant, Marc?"

"There is a 90 percent chance you'll need it in the next two years. We'll know in plenty of time because you will slowly experience congestive heart failure and become progressively more tired."

I have spent six months being tired, barely alive only in the morning. You mean there is more-tired-than-this?

"I don't want someone else's heart, Marc. I like mine."

He looks like he's about to say something, then stops with a wan smile.

I perk up. "You're being a sober doctor telling me the worst case so I won't be disappointed if it does happen, right?"

"There's a little of that because I know you can handle it. I didn't want to raise the topic again until you'd experienced a summer of recovery and I'd seen your numbers. I'd be very surprised if you could avoid a transplant, though. Your lungs and other organs are doing yeoman's work, making up for the failure of your left ventricle. But they can't do this forever and will eventually protest. I will not list you yet, of course, because I'd be laughed out of my profession; you are doing amazingly well with what you have. Watch for unusual fatigue and shortness of breath. Let me know immediately."

We walk slowly back to the car in silence, seeking shelter in the darkness of the garage. "They've taken away all my hope," Jack finally says as we pay our parking fee. We are just like other people who leave MGH every day in altered states, fumbling for change and a polite smile for the attendant.

In spite of our devastation, we had to concede Marc's sensitivity in not raising the T-word during a fragile summer when we had needed to believe in fairies. Now all the facts were in and we approached the future soberly. I'd become a statistic, one of the cardiac patients whose EF does not improve. Jack and I spiraled into depression. He suffered more than I did, I think. He looked terrible, like the flu was coming on.

I'd never known despair before. I'd always been able to figure a way out of a bad situation. Most unfortunately for our weaver friend Ann, we visited her in southern New Hampshire, as planned, on our way home to Maine. The mother of one of my dearest friends, she is like a mother to me and she'd been worried sick. The plan had been to delight her with how well I looked and with the good news we had expected.

Instead, we arrived a shipwreck.

Always a bustler, Ann went into high gear over the next few weeks, sending me encouraging notes and quotations. I needed every word of love, and yet it felt like judgment, too, as though I was not allowed to fall apart. Ann had faced her breast cancer battle with fortitude and cheer—at least that's the face she had showed to me—and had been rewarded with more than twenty years of vibrant health. Yet I knew I needed more time before I could rally.

I wrote Ann a white-lie letter—a defense my grandmother had taught me to employ only when feelings were at stake and the lie would do no harm—assuring her that I was chipper. The frantic letters subsided. Now I could retreat and deal privately with a normal reaction to devastating news without feeling the need to prop up anyone else besides Jack and me. I felt badly for alarming Ann. My devastation was a storm that simply needed to run its course.

I called my matter-of-fact sister Callie, knowing that with her I could unravel safely. She reminded me that everyone had always known about the transplant—even Jack. Oh, well. The denial was great while it lasted.

Jack returned to Boston for a week of work and I was once again in that dentist's chair Dad always evoked, dealing with my future by myself. One morning, when I got Jack's usual seven-o'clock phone call, I told him exactly what I'd been thinking about since dawn: I suddenly understood suicide as an option for some people. I had never before considered my own suicide, as I had never before believed in my own death. I was not suicidal, I assured him, simply newly respectful of those who chose that path.

On other mornings I'd wake and see strung across my bedroom window a spiderweb lit with early-morning dew like a tiny silver Ferris wheel, confirming that dark thoughts had no chance against life. November was a good teacher. If you take the time to look, on a misty, gray November day, the firs are always greener and the lingering leaves more golden.

37

THE URGE TO HOLD TONI'S HAND is overwhelming. Having massaged my body back to life for a few months now, she's decided that it's time for me to pitch in. So here we are at my first yoga class since I stretched for release and the heavens piled onto my chest. I've been dreaming of this terrifying bliss since I took my first steps in the hospital, hamstrings tight as cords. In spite of my fear, I am longing to stretch deeply enough to feel my spine loosen and energy course through my body, to experience the quieting of my mind from yoga's discipline.

I grip the handrail and pull myself up the steep, creaking stairs to the "ballroom," a former town dance hall now used for movement classes of all kinds, a large space that smells of meetings, bake sales, bean suppers, and sweat from the previous dance class. No one else seems to notice. I need fresh air desperately and am too weak to open one of the huge windows, too guilty to ask Toni to do one more thing for me. The frustration is suffocating.

I feel very shy with the other women. They greet each other with the easy camaraderie of friends at an old-fashioned potluck supper, hugging and cooing. Toni gently leads me into the circle and gets me a mat. The creaking floor, the smell of oiled wood and a century of bodies gathering here, the light the color of weak tea, my fear—everything takes me back to kindergarten in the basement of the Congregational church and the feeling of crossing a dangerous threshold. When Toni sits next to me on her own mat and turns to another woman to say hello, I want to run after my mother and beg her to take me home. But I am a big girl now and I know this is good for me. Time to get back in the saddle.

The instructor leads the class in easy, familiar poses, and my stiff body gradually stretches like a cat feeling the sun. Then she asks us to lie on our backs with our knees up.

"Now roll your knees to the floor on your right. Keep your arms straight out at shoulder height, shoulders relaxed into the floor."

Toni's eyebrows ask whether I am okay. She knows this twist is similar to the pose I was in when the vise began to tighten in my chest. *Will it happen again? Did the pose tear my artery and unleash the clot?* I gaze up at the high ceiling as though it is heaven and hold Toni in the corner of one eye to keep me on earth, breathing my way into the pose until I am there.

Nothing happens.

I am stiff, but it is the stiffness of disuse. I keep breathing evenly to relax my body as I go more deeply into the pose, releasing my hips and lower back, opening my chest. My friend has just given me another gift.

As November continued its quiet progress toward winter, I became more and more aware of my life force—what Buddhists call *prana*—returning to my body. I felt it in my improved balance, the strength of my voice, the confident way my fingers held a toothbrush. I believed that my physical training plan deserved lots of credit. The exercise, yoga, massage, and cranial osteopathy were doing what they were supposed to do: finding the health inherent in my body and inviting it to thrive again.

I added a monthly acupuncture treatment, on pure faith. After each appointment, I felt relaxed, my energy evened out, but I had no idea whether it was doing any real good. My faith was well founded, it turns out. In November 2001 at the annual meeting of the American Heart Association, researchers announced that they had proved that acupuncture dramatically helps people with high blood pressure and severe heart problems. The research, conducted by doctors at the University of California School of Medicine in Los Angeles, demonstrated that the ancient Chinese practice has the potential to reduce pressure on the heart.

It didn't matter to me that from the point of view of many Western doctors, the jury was still out on the effectiveness of most "alternative treatments." I was taking control, and my study of one was yielding results: I had been freezing all summer, yet as the season grew colder, I began to blaze.

"Oooooh, you feel so good and toasty today!" Judy hums as she bends over me on her osteopathic table.

"When you first came here, you were so cold, so brittle," she muses, almost to herself, as she pokes and pulls here and there until I feel the blood flowing through my body and my cheeks glow pink.

"My goal is to get you into a state of warm chocolate pudding."

Warm chocolate pudding. Now there is a goal.

Her gushing makes me feel as though I have finally succeeded at the high jump. When I was thirteen, I ran pell-mell for the sandpit, then lost my nerve, kicked the pole, and kept on running—failing gym and disgracing myself. Even winning the prize for the eighth-grade essay contest didn't make up for the humiliation. I resolve in Judy's office that this time I'm going to sail right over the pole. I'm going for the warm chocolate pudding.

On Judy's wall, watching over our search for health in my body, was a large sepia-toned print of a Rubens Madonna. Looking at her sad, almond-shaped eyes and Mona Lisa smile, I began to think about what Christianity and spirituality meant to me, now that my life had changed so dramatically. It was inevitable. When the body is weak and you have become pure spirit, your first instinct is to call on whatever spiritual training you had as a child. For me, that was the Catholic religion, even though I hadn't always seen it as a great haven of spirituality. My ambivalence had been clear even in the hospital, when I refused Communion from a small, gentle bird of an old lady. She came to my room offering a chalice I knew would be filled with hosts, the body of Christ, and when I declined, she backed away quickly with a bow. I hadn't meant to chase her away. I had been polite, and a little sad, even. I knew that the gods had gotten me through this, but I was not ready to give credit to any specific one. I needed time to think.

I had always believed in a Great Spirit. I called it Love. Plato called it The Good. When I first read Plato in college, I became a fan because The Good hit a happier, larger note closer to my beliefs than the idea of a punishing God waiting in the confessional to smite me for my sins.

"Bless me, father, for I have sinned. It has been one week since my last confession. I lost my temper three times." *It was Callie's fault anyhow. She was bugging me.*

I hesitated to call The Good, this Great Spirit that I felt, God because too often God was a hostage of extremists whose true gods seemed to be Fear and Control. Organized religion had always felt confining to me, a box surrounding something—the spirit—that simply couldn't be contained. With a box, you are either in or out. If you are out, you perish in the Bermuda Triangle, the opening to hell, as Lil explained to me, or you are labeled as an "infidel." These attitudes have led to wars in ancient times as well as in our own, all in the name of God.

I worshipped Spirit daily at sunsets and sunrises, when I went walking in the hills, when I saw frost etch my windows in the morning sun. Literature was my chapel for contemplating truths, as was our dinner table filled with friends bearing gifts of insight and mirth. For me, life was the sacrament.

The entire time I was unconscious, I felt a great love surrounding me like a ball of warm, coddling light. Others at death's threshold have described this same sensation of energy. I took it as a sign that despite all my unruly beliefs, God is love and he loves me. This was what we had recited in catechism at St. Mary's parish and I believed it.

Finally ready to consider spirituality in the context of all that had happened, I was open to another of Toni's gentle nudges. In late November, as I left our massage session, she gave me a set of taped lectures by Caroline Myss, Ph.D., author of *Anatomy of the Spirit* and a respected figure in holistic medicine. Toni told me to listen to them out of order, last one first, because my impatient brain would want the conclusion. Only then was I to listen to the tape on the fourth chakra, love.

38

As Jack's wheels crunch down the driveway and back to Boston on this drizzly November Monday morning, I dutifully slip in the tape Toni recommended. According to the flyer, Caroline Myss sees healing as a fusion of Eastern and Western spiritual and medical traditions, which seems to me a sensible embrace in our shrinking world. I am intrigued by her suggestion that healing is a mix of the secular and the divine, that the ultimate goal of being one with the Spirit, of becoming whole, is shared by Christianity, Buddhism, and Judaism, as well as Eastern and enlightened Western medicine.

Dr. Myss asserts that in the beginning the world was energy and therefore so are we. Was this why I felt warmth as I hid deep within my body in the hospital? Had I returned to my beginning? Because the alignment of the energetic and the physical is so strong, she believes that we have the potential to heal ourselves, drawing on the spirit, with a little help from allopathic and complementary medicine.

She has my attention immediately. In my diminished state, I know that I am all energy. This is why the sick feel like ghosts of themselves. We *are*. Matter goes first during disease, but our spirit, our energy, lingers—as witnessed by the anesthesiologists I kicked in the operating room when I should have been dead.

If we are first and last energy, then every decision we make either recharges or drains the energy we are born with. Human energy is like a bank account, she says, with a finite amount of money in it. You put money in or take it out. Squandering cash can drain our account, as we know from bounced checks. So, we have to learn to stop the withdrawals from our energy bank that leave us spiritually empty, drained of energy, and vulnerable to disease.

Once I had great energy. I remember what it felt like to walk swiftly, to skip and skate, to talk and laugh and not need a nap. Any one of those actions seems like a miracle now.

As I lie in bed with the tape recorder clicking, my mind drifts and I see myself in an airport, hauling bags and racing for a plane, pale and exhausted. I see a business colleague coyly remarking that there are givers and takers in this world, and I realize now that this was fair warning. I see myself during a stormy blackout, desperately wrapping family Christmas presents by candlelight, presents that could never fill the empty spaces in our relationships. I remember how sick I was before the heart attack. And now I knew why. I had bankrupted my spirit.

My attention drifts back to the voice on the tape. I learn that intuition is the greatest of energetic forces. If we harness it and put it to work for us, says Myss, intuition has the potential to heal.

This is great news. You cannot be successful in sales without great intuition, so I figure I already possess a tool I can use to replenish the energy I have lost. It's a tool I have already begun to use, I realize. Intuition brought me to Mount Auburn Hospital, to Maine, to Toni and Judy and my cardiac rehab program. It sent me to a psychiatrist, who let me cry until I was cleansed and open to a deeper understanding of my broken heart. My intuition even rejected the taste of coffee in the morning and a martini before dinner.

The sound of the lake rippling from gusts of chill wind rouses me out of my head and into the day. I decide to delay listening to the tape on the fourth chakra, love. I pull on my sweats for a walk, get my foot stuck in the elastic, and crash into the bedpost. I can feel the bruise rising. Damn blood thinners.

My house arrest at this spare, increasingly dark time of year, offered the quiet I needed to discover what drained me of precious energy. I began my research simply, by paying attention. Without the strong body that had deluded me into thinking I could handle anything, I had the opportunity to practice being in the moment, to simply notice.

I first noticed my reaction to large and obvious energy drains: crowds, loud and multilayered conversation, children running in circles, a squawking television, pleasantries with shop clerks or strangers, loud noises and flashing lights, the slightest violence or tension in a movie, and multitask moments like talking on the phone while stirring a pot and listening to news on the radio. I had been too busy and strong to notice the drain of noisy, normal life. Now a slight tightening of the muscles in the corners of my eyes signaled that I was becoming exhausted. I paid attention to it and retreated quickly, if I could.

Often Jack saw the look in my eyes before I could even feel it and would gracefully walk me out of a gathering after thirty minutes or declare nap time when someone knocked on our door. We accepted no invitations to dinner; talking and eating at the same time were still among my most challenging activities. Jack performed all our errands.

The few times I went out—to the post office or the grocery store—I was struck by how tiring the simple act of popping in and out of a car could be.

It surprised those close to me, but I did not struggle with my dependence on Jack. It was delightful. As Lil said, stopping the vacuum, the thought in midair like dust suddenly apparent in a ray of sun, "Do you realize that this is the first time in your marriage that you have been together for more than a long weekend or a vacation?" She startled me with that one.

Jack's solid devotion became the raft from which I dove to the bottom of my soul to see what I might find.

We are alone for Thanksgiving and content in our separateness because we feel wanted by our families. At last. For years Thanksgiving had marked the beginning of the season of anguish, silence, and distance. This year we are alone by choice, since travel is too much for me, and a houseful of guests—no matter how helpful—is unimaginable. The difference is that this year we are free to say "I love you" on the phone and have it reciprocated with no reservations, no embarrassment. Our families' expressiveness is rebuilding my trust, releasing me from yearning—a true drain on the spirit, as anyone who has ever experienced unrequited love knows.

Even without guests, we have prepared enough food for ten people, cooking with our hearts, not our heads. Steam from glistening dishes of pureed roasted squash, green peas, and bitter turnip mingles with candle smoke. The organic turkey is roasted nut-brown and bursting with stuffing. Jack has made his famous mashed potatoes with the skins on and butter and raw onions and I am going to eat a large dollop, so there.

As we slowly enjoy our private feast, the late-afternoon sun throws slanted golden light into the dining room until it glows like the inside of Cinderella's pumpkin. We laugh and cry together and toast the gods, grateful for their compassion and generosity. Besides the obvious reasons to be thankful, we joke about having avoided my sister Leesa's flavorless turkey stuffing, made just the way my family has always liked it: straight out of the bag with water and an egg. Of course they would argue that mine is just too-too, with onions, apples, celery, and all those exotic-sounding herbs. Laughing wickedly, irreverently, makes us feel normal. We know that out at Leesa's house on Cape Elizabeth, my family is doing the same thing: "The chestnuts were bad enough, but do you remember the year she stuffed it with *oysters*?"

WINTER

39

JACK AND I blow through his eldest daughter's front door, our arms filled with presents, chill air and snow flurries at our back. Small tow-headed children greet us, eyes lit like Christmas bulbs. An onlooker would take it for a scene from a Victorian Christmas card.

The reality is less picturesque. The children know that their grand-father Jack is divorced from their grandmother Brenda. Their mother, Mary Kate, is wracked with pain from rheumatoid arthritis. Their father, Walter, commutes to New York City to support the household and is home only on weekends. And this is grandfather Jack's second wife's first big outing since emergency open-heart surgery.

By Hallmark standards, we are a family wreck.

Mary Kate and Walter have instructed the children that they must be quiet, quiet, quiet. Jack has sternly warned me, too. Impossible for any of us! We barely saw them over the summer because I was simply too weak for child energy, so within minutes I am snuggling Jack's grandchildren like puppies, hoping none of them has a cold. I have been warned to avoid crowds and children; with half a heart, I am vulnerable to infection.

Simon sneezes on my hands. Jack tenses.

To hell with caution! Here I am with a boisterous, germ-spewing *crowd* of children, defying the gods. Then Fiona nudges seven-year-old Wally, who steps forward with something on his mind, on all their minds.

"Deborah, may we see your scars?" They giggle, as though about to put their hands into spaghetti brains on Halloween.

It is a dangerous moment. Waffling and excuses will not do for intent and curious children. I decide that a simple display without the squeamishness I truly feel is the best course, so I peel my sweater off my left shoulder to reveal the ICD slit and the hard edges of the box beneath my skin.

Their eyes are big.

"May I touch it?" asks Wally, of course.

Once he is through, grinning triumphantly, tauntingly at Fiona and Simon, they approach with trembling extended fingers. Then Sean has to have a turn, too. When they have survived the touch, they look at each other.

"And here's the scar down the center of my chest."

I pull the neck of my sweater down. The upper part of the scar is healing quite nicely, so this is the least-scary display. They won't know that I am showing only part of the truth. Four blond heads come close, studying my chest with the seriousness of surgeons.

"And then here's the scar on my leg." I unzip my pants and show them the red gash along the inside of my right thigh. This one gets them.

"Uuughh! Why do you have a scar there?"

"This is where they took out a healthy vein to bypass the bad one. The good vein is now sewn onto my heart." Silence. This takes a lot of thought. It's taken the last six months of thought for me, so I give them time.

"Deborah," says Wally again. They press forward, so close I could gather them up like a bunch of flowers. "We just want you to know that we're awfully glad you're not dead."

Children are often the sensible ones. When my nephew Chris caught Callie crying one night after she returned home from the hospital, he put his hand on her arm and peered into her eyes, shaking her to get her attention.

"Mum. Mum." She looked up at him through a waterfall. "Is she still breathing, Mum," he probed. It was more of a statement than a question, a finding of fact.

And he was right. I *was* still breathing, and that was the important thing. Laughter jump-started her lungs and Callie resumed breathing herself.

* * *

I am sitting on the couch, eyes closed, rigid with anticipation.

"Don't peek!" Jack hollers when he sees an eyelash flutter. I can tell from his voice that he is above me. Somewhere. What is he *doing*?

"Open your eyes *now*."

I follow orders and look tentatively around the living room. There in the corner is our Christmas tree, sparkling with ornaments we have collected over the years. Beneath it are gaily wrapped presents from me to Jack, newspaper-wrapped presents from Jack to me.

"Damn," I hear above me.

I look toward his voice and find him standing with one leg on the back of the couch and one on an upholstered arm, reaching for the ceiling beams. And then I see it: THE BUG, dangling in the air like an entangled parachute jumper.

"Oh, this would have been so good! I blew it!"

Jack has rigged a belay that was supposed to work at the flick of his finger, sending the big, ugly, black plastic bug down in front of my face when I opened my eyes.

"So that's what you've been practicing all day in here!"

Both entrances to the living room are hung with signs: DO NOT ENTER. THIS MEANS YOU.

The Bug has been a part of our life ever since Jack first packed it into a small box and anonymously sent it to me at my father's house during our courtship. Dad opened the package, not realizing that it was not addressed to him, and had to steady himself against a wall, laughing. Grasping immediately what the sender had intended, he placed it on the threshold of my old bedroom to shock me, successfully, when I arrived for our weekend visit. I knew then that Jack and Dad would get along just fine.

Since then, the receiver of The Bug has the next year in which to startle the other—and the contest is escalating. A month before my heart attack, I had a chef hide it on a covered silver platter to be delivered ceremoniously as dessert. It's unclear who was more surprised, Jack or the dutiful, humorless waiter.

In adjusting to my new life, I have forgotten about The Bug. But

Jack hasn't. He is the consummate survivor. As a boy he learned to keep his room neat while his father threw lamps in a drunken rage below, to climb his Everest—the snow-covered coal pile in the backyard—when a storm was brewing inside his home. It was early training for a life well lived. Jack knows how to survive in an alpine whiteout, how to build a snow cave against the deafening wind, how to turn ice into hot tea, and how to rescue a shaky Christmas with laughter.

The day after Christmas, my father and sisters arrived for dinner and an overnight visit. They had hesitated to come because they knew how hard it was for me not to take on the role of hostess and to allow myself to receive help, a requirement of my new social life.

They emerged from their cars with tentative steps, smiles pasted on like stickers, shoulders hunched as if to tread more lightly. Dad looked unusually frail to me; my illness had walloped him. But all of a sudden the fake smile disappeared and he grinned widely, looking me up and down in happy disbelief. He had purposely stayed away, letting my sisters visit and report back to him, because he was too afraid of what he would see. He preferred to hear my voice getting stronger and stronger in our phone calls. To see me now was to believe that I really was who my voice had promised. He gave me flowers and fussed at me to sit down, at the same time delighting in my serving him tea and his favorite homemade ginger cookies.

As I put the finishing touches on our dinner, my sisters hovered like dragonflies, darting in and out of the kitchen. Then we went upstairs, dressed in sparkles and silk, and came back down looking stunning because we were happy. *Why couldn't it always have been like this?* I pushed away thoughts of the previous Christmas, when it had been so emotionally complicated to be together that in the end we chose to be apart. I understood the reasons, but at the time I had been hurt and impatient. My impatience had probably contributed to their distance. But now they were here. I tried to be calm in my joy, but it was difficult for me to behave with restraint in a moment this happy.

I also felt tension registering in the skin around my eyes from so many family members watching my every move and begging me to sit down. I had become used to my small, solitary life in the kitchen with my alarm watch—pacing myself, learning what I could do and could not do, monitored by Jack alone. All these guardians made things more exhausting than if I had proceeded quietly on my own. But I didn't know that yet. I noticed the tension the way you notice a bee buzz harmlessly over the picnic table, only to remember the moment later, after you have been stung.

At dinner, I asked Jack to get me a tissue from the kitchen. A simple thing. I thought I was being cooperative. Everyone wanted me to stop popping up from the table, and they were right because it did tire me. But it is one thing to ask for help when you are too weak to move from your bed; it takes a much larger effort to speak up when you have pale roses in your cheeks and you have just cooked a savory pumpkin and rosemary lasagna with chicken sausage. It's hard not to feel like a fraud. Still, I was tired.

Jack was talking with Ann and they were laughing uproariously. It had been such a long time since we'd heard laughter like that in this house. So I guiltily asked again. And again.

"Just a second," Jack chortled, hand on mine and eyes on Ann as she finished her story.

I had lost their attention for just a moment in their long vigil, and in that moment lost my life-support. I heard myself begin to scream—desperate, old screams that shattered the windows and brought in frigid air.

"All I want is a tissue and not only will you not let me get it myself, no one will get it for me. What the hell am I supposed to do?"

Everything went blinding white and I heard my voice from the years following my mother's death, a time of great aloneness when I had tried to keep her alive in the wilting birthday cakes I baked from Duncan Hines mixes, tried my flawed best to keep watch over my sisters and brother. *You tell me not to boss you around. Then why won't you just pick up your room, clear the table, empty the dishwasher, take out the garbage? Why won't anybody help me? I have homework.*

Silence. When I could see again, I fled to the bathroom to hide my shame and to compose myself.

William Faulkner wrote, "The past is never dead. It's not even past." Does heartbreak ever leave the body? Perhaps it's like mercury spilled from a broken thermometer, tiny silver globules escaping into cracks and corners, never fully cleaned up no matter how hard we try.

I didn't know how to come out of the bathroom; I was so ashamed, so confused at the rage that I had spilled all over our table, rage that had no place here anymore.

With time I've come to view this incident as a strange sign of progress. In light moments, I refer to it as my spiritual heart's osteopathic moment. After Judy prods my body in her treatments, sometimes I am sore for a couple of days. It used to scare me, or cause me to doubt my progress or her skill. But I've learned that these are typical results of homeopathic therapies. With the release of blockages, the healthy processes of the body acquire more and more space within the body. As health begins to reoccupy its rightful place, disease is displaced. The process of displacement may be a painful one, presenting itself as a headache, stiffness, dizziness, a slight cold. But, when the blockage is finally cleared, sometimes with a little more help from Judy, I always feel immediate relief. It took months of patient work before Judy could sense my fascia untwist from the surgery's trauma, and we will continue to work together to ease the inevitable blockages that arise from simply living. I can no longer handle dams in my body.

If this is true of the body, why not of the soul, especially if that soul has experienced trauma? Why can't an ugly outburst indicate sadness heading for the exit, creating a clearing in the healing heart so that love will have more room? I was certainly right on schedule. Patients suffering from postoperative depression typically emerge from it after about six months.

When I returned to the table, a box of tissues was by my place and faces were glowing with tenderness—and looking as baffled as they must have looked during my adolescent storms, when I couldn't see my siblings as the children they were because I didn't realize that I was a child, too.

Dad squeezed my hand and the party resumed. I felt horrible and apologized, but we didn't need to talk about it. Intuitively, Jack and my family knew that wherever I'd gone in my head, I had to go there alone. At the halfway mark, with a new year peeking around the corner, this incident was far from the setback I took it for at the time. I was becoming whole.

40

JACK STAYED HOME for the first two weeks of January. It was his boss, Henri's, idea; Jack needed a deep rest. Since I was past crisis, it would be a real vacation for Jack during his favorite season of long, frigid nights and white days. But winter had other plans.

On January 7 it began to rain, then to sleet, then to hail, and carried on like that for two days, finally freezing into a sparkling fairyland of crystal. The reality was frightening: trees were bent to the ground or brutally toppled altogether, power lines came crashing down and lay across roads twitching and spitting sparks, pumps no longer delivered water from wells, and anyone without a wood stove had no heat. The storm darkened 750,000 homes before it was done. Ice coated every tree like a candied apple. The air crackled as temperatures plummeted. In some places, the wind chill factor was twenty below. People were terrified of the wind, because when it roared through, whole trees snapped and fell or treetops blew off and exploded like bombs into a thousand pieces. As ice shivered through the sky, the air filled with the continuous din of glass shattering.

It was the ice storm of 1998, a month of endurance that Mainers will remember for decades.

Our town was at the heart of the storm for New England. Trucks with linemen from states as far away as Hawaii rolled down Main Street painted with MAINE OR BUST on their doors. The town cheered them like a liberating army. CNN and other television networks moved in to cover the siege live from the grocery store parking lot, reporters turning up their collars as ice pummeled them. Maine Public Radio broadcast a survival talk show. We listened to it on our scratchy transistor radio every night in our candlelit house and felt as though the whole state were one small united community—a rare occurrence, since Mainers are an opinionated and ornery lot. The storm brought us back to a time when people both needed each other and no one.

Jack and I were without power for eight days. He knew that I grew cold easily and that our woodpile would only last a week. Our phone lines had been pulled down by a tree that had fallen into our swamp, which meant that my alarm watch, which transmitted through the telephone, was now useless. If I needed to be transported to a hospital, an ambulance could not get to us—a huge old pine lay across the driveway. The town hospital was out of electrical power for days, too, operating on generators. But evacuating me to Portland to be near Maine Medical Center was impossible. We would have been in even more danger on the road. This was exactly the isolation that my doctors had feared. I hoped they were too busy to follow the news.

Before the danger even dawned on me, Jack's survival instincts had kicked in and he embarked on what can only be called a rescue mission. First he used his cell phone, while it still had power, to reach Cookie, the tree guy. Cookie's strapping sons came over to clear our driveway ahead of other pressing requests. In minutes, that old pine was cut into tractor-wheel chunks and pushed to the side of the road like discarded children's blocks.

After getting his own generator working for Arlene and the children, Joe was the first to come down the cleared driveway. He reattached our electrical power lines for when the juice got switched on again, hauled our telephone pole up from where it had toppled into the frozen swamp, and—without asking for New England Telephone's blessing—restored power to our phone. Bob came down the driveway next, his chest-length beard covered with ice instead of sawdust. He had brought wood just in case our old pile was rotten. As the days wore on, our driveway became a throughway of concern. As Joe once said politely, "Deb, I hope you don't mind my sayin', but you and Jack are not exactly what I'd call 'handy' people," and everybody knew it.

We were one of the lucky families. We had a gas cooking stove, two wood stoves, and town water, so we did not suffer the consequences of a frozen well pump. Jack began to deliver water to our neighbors, and as word went out people came to us with pans and buckets. It was flu season, and I kept a constant pot of soup on the stove, doling it out for visitors to take home in large yogurt containers. At one point, I tried to give a pot of soup to the town shelter, but I learned that it was against government regulations. Their soup had to come from a can.

One day our friend Hartley, who can fix anything, came by and I offered him some homemade pita bread, hot off the griddle. The rolled-up bread looked like a sixth finger on his hands, the size of scored hams. He stood with me watching the chickadees and woolly woodpeckers peck frantically at our suet feeder, their feathers so fluffed up that they looked stuffed. He told me that what he missed most about losing his hearing was listening to the chickadees when he goes hunting. I tried not to think too long about Hartley hunting with no hearing in the first place.

Those eight days were like being transported back to a bygone time. We lived with the light, up at sunrise and retiring by four-thirty, when the world went black. Jack split and hauled wood every day, all day, returning slimy with sweat. I boiled water to wash dishes and Jack by candlelight. We slept on the first floor by the fireplace for warmth and ease in tending the stove, but also because, if a tree fell, we would be safest near the chimney, which might withstand the blow. Jack was up all night feeding the stove to prevent the pipes from bursting, and in the total darkness we listened for a telltale crack as trees swayed and hissed above. One morning I spent an hour cleaning Jack's grandmother's wooden coffee grinder and surprised him with a hot cup of bitter brew laced with scrapings of frozen cream stored in our makeshift refrigerator, a bank of snow.

Al's hardware store became the town gathering place. As the storm progressed, Jack bolted first thing each morning for the place where men holding steaming cups hung around and traded information, wearing one-piece mustard-colored Dickey work suits and blaze-orange caps pushed back on their foreheads. It was here that they learned who'd gotten power and who had none yet, who was in trouble, who had what equipment. Al stepped up delivery and the hardware floor was heaped with boxes of survival tools—kerosene, motor oil, large plastic gas containers, candles, batteries.

One early morning Jack came upon a caravan of carpetbaggers

who had just parked their loaded pickups at Al's, bringing kerosene lamps, chain saws, and generators. He made fast friends with the generator salesman and came home before 9 A.M. with the biggest generator he could put on his credit card. That night the temperature dipped especially low and the generator saved us from frozen pipes.

Jack blossomed during the crisis. Though he was exhausted, I saw the satisfaction in the way he swaggered into the kitchen smeared with grime and wood chips, proud of real labor. By keeping the house warm, the driveway clear, and the phone working, Jack lessened the feelings of helplessness that had haunted him since May. He was saving me with his own hands.

Jack's vacation ended and he returned to Boston. He always looked gray in the early Monday morning light as he packed his bag for the week, as though he were holding his breath until Thursday evening. He buried himself in his work, spending long hours at the office, often continuing with business dinners to fill time. As he wandered corporate corridors throughout the day, he faithfully, obsessively called to let me know his whereabouts.

"Hi, love. It's Jack," he'd say on the answering machine, as if I'd forgotten the sound of his voice. "I'm leaving the office now for a haircut around the corner. I'll have my beeper on. I'll call you again when I get back. Then I'm going to my other office in Framingham. I'll call you when I get in the car so you'll know where I am." He was like the weatherman, announcing every shift in the prevailing winds.

When he had no evening obligations, he was in bed early, on my schedule, seeking synchronization. We'd talk by phone about nothing at all, sometimes just listening to each other breathe before falling asleep, a rope stretched taut between us.

On the western shore of the lake, a large light kept me company. Some nights I watched videos of foreign films sent by my cousin Anne, who knows Jack hates subtitles. They were my secret stash of chocolates under the pillow. But mainly I read until I felt sleepy. I discovered the pleasures, and the comedy, of books on gardening. Gardening writers opine with such authority about nature, a force that will not be ruled. No mention of ice storms in their tidy world of cooperative or naughty plants. One author declared the hydrangea—an innocent bush with as much right to flourish as any other—vulgar. I determined to plant a few more around the house, aware that I was anticipating spring, thinking in the future tense.

Since autumn, our friends Fritz and Brian had been asking me to come for an early dinner to break up a week when I was alone. Whether I was the guest or not, mind you, the dinner would still have been at five-thirty. That was the way we lived in western Maine in winter, when the sky was black. No one found it odd that wild parties ended at eight and we went to bed when most people were beginning dinner.

Perhaps emboldened by the ice storm, I accepted the invitation when Fritz called again in late January, and Brian picked me up in pitch darkness at five. I took off my alarm watch and left it on the floor of the foyer, where I would be sure to see it after my furlough. It was snowing lightly and our headlights searched the lacy blackness for the road as we dipped and rose to the next town, and then bumped up the steep hill to their white farmhouse.

Fritz was busy in the kitchen. Fussing, serious. Tiny turkey chicks had just hatched and were wobbling around in a box on the floor under warming lights. Clocks ticked. Candles flickered. New friends joined us and the conversation soared. The meal, poached salmon and vegetables, was beautifully and thoughtfully prepared. Fritz reigned at the head of the table as I imagined his baronial ancestors had once in Bavarian castles. Brian played his practiced role of charming foil to the crusty good man he'd loved for thirty-three years. I drank wine—two whole glasses.

The ride home through the darkness was as thrilling as a final run on a toboggan. I had ventured out of the house at night, past my normal bedtime, in the snow, without Jack. I had met new people and drunk wine. I had even worn perfume.

At other times my confidence would slide, one time quite literally. It happened when I ventured a ten-minute solo drive into town in my little red car. After driving the whole way in second gear and parking beside the bank, I made my way on an icy path through the hedges to the ATM machine. Suddenly my feet flew out from under me and I lay gasping on the ground. I began to cry from the shock. Would the box fire? How bad would the bruise be? Was I hemorrhaging? I unraveled in broad daylight, on the cold ice, right next to the bushes.

And then I realized that I was not alone. A large, doughy teenage boy was peering down at me, having just come out of the ATM booth. He stared at me dully, as though I were a ship passing on some distant horizon.

"I'm so sorry. I just fell. I'm not well. I'm on a lot of drugs. I'm not allowed to fall . . . My heart . . ." I fumbled with the words, embarrassed at being caught bawling like a big baby.

He just looked down at me, impassive. I struggled to my feet alone.

Once I had cleared his way and he'd sullenly lumbered through, I felt angry at his callousness. Then I reconsidered. It was a good lesson to have learned within the safety of my own town. If I intended to venture forth into the world outside my bedroom, I had to remember that it was not always a gentle place.

41

UP FOR A WEEKEND OF SKIING in early February, my nephew Chris pads into my study to watch me write this book. Of course, I cannot write with a twelve-year-old boy straining to see every word over my shoulder. Then I realize that he has another agenda.

Chris sits on the couch and asks thoughtfully in his low, quiet voice, "Deborah, do they know why you had the heart attack?"

"No, love, no one knows."

Then he looks straight into my eyes. It is clear that he has wanted to say something for a long time and that nothing is going to get in his way.

"Maybe you loved too many people and your heart got so full it had to break."

The world stops. I retreat into my body and peer out from behind my skin. Hours or seconds later I return to the room.

While Chris sees nothing amiss, I feel as though a dam is threatening to burst inside me. I mumble something about how I like that image and will keep it as a present from him. My acceptance is enough for Chris, a child like any other, whose daily, earth-shattering insights come as naturally as breathing. He wanders off, leaving me stunned. *Was it my particular brand of love that caused my heart to break?*

A child of twelve, if loved, has not yet learned what he should not say because it is too truthful. So I took Chris's question into my soul. It had lingered from my first conscious moments in the hospital, a face reflected in the bottom of a stream, an echo I heard only when alone. While my body went about winter days—of cold hands and swelling bruises the size of eggs, fear of hemorrhaging from a spill on the icy driveway, dizzy spells as I made my way in the dark to the bathroom, and a left arm still frozen tight from scar tissue—my mind continued to explore *why* my heart had broken. In August I had blamed others or myself; now therapy and reflection had cured me of such useless and dishonest behavior. They say that when the student is ready, a teacher appears. I was ready to listen to Caroline Myss's tape on the fourth chakra, love. It corresponds with the Christian fourth sacrament, marriage, and the Jewish fourth sefira, beauty.

Echoing my mother's wisdom and catechism's teachings, Dr. Myss reminded me that love has two sides: both giving and forgiving. I've always had the giving part down pat. I was the giver of gifts, time, meals, conversation, of kindnesses and pleasantries. It was natural to me, a habit I saw no point in breaking because it led to trust, satisfaction, and joy. Yet it had also led to disappointment and exhaustion.

Listening to the Myss tape, I had a hunch that the drain of energy that had made me ill in the months before my heart attack was related to the forgiving part. But what is forgiveness?

I approached the question by thinking first about what made me feel hurt. What prompted a need for forgiveness in the first place? I concluded that I had always been extraordinarily sensitive to people who withhold love—meaning kindness, affection, thoughtfulness, fairness, honesty, courtesy, compassion, effort, generosity, and communication. In a sense, I have always bruised easily. Withholders have perplexed and sometimes angered me—a waste of precious emotion, since the world is full of people who withhold love for all kinds of reasons, both intentional and unintentional. People withhold love because of politics, fear, ignorance, preoccupation, cunning, selfishness, self-protectiveness, sadness, or because they think someone doesn't need it—someone like me, the independent one, the leader.

After many late-night and kitchen-sink talks with Jack, I realized that at the core of my particular brand of hurt was a betrayal of trust. Betrayal does not have to be monumental, though the word sounds epic. We face small, draining betrayals of trust every day. Consider a trip to the store for milk. Knowing full well that you probably shouldn't, you trust that the cashier will take your money nicely, give you change, and say "thank you," that it will be a simple, pleasant transaction. Instead the cashier is sullen. She mumbles. She doesn't look at you. "Thank you" goes unsaid. Betrayal may sound like too dramatic a word to use for such a mundane exchange. But even minor betrayals sap vital energy and the cumulative effect can be devastating.

Some people deal with betrayal better than others. I am not one of them. On my first day of grammar school, Dad watched me skip down our dirt road to the bus stop—ponytail whipping back and forth, tin lunch box whack-whacking my skinny white legs—and remembered praying, "Please be good to her. She gets so disappointed." Way back then, he knew what my life's work would be.

Jack has a great trick, born of too much experience with betrayal. When his trust is violated, he can usually stop the energy drain by imagining softly puffing the hurt away, like blowing out a candle.

My friend Juliana once advised, "People who are in great pain themselves often do not know that they are inflicting pain on another person. They are suffering too much to realize their impact." Maybe my nephew Chris was right: I had taken too many people into my heart without fully accepting their *humanity*, their capacity to disappoint. Just like me. Perhaps this acceptance of humanity was forgiveness, the other half of love.

On a lark years ago, I had gone to a psychic, who told me that I had been a man in most past lives and had come into this life a woman to learn more about love. At the time I found it amusing. (Frankly, if I am here to learn anything, I would rather it be about love than, say, mathematics or taxidermy.) Shortly thereafter I met Jack and discovered the infinite bliss of tucking clean socks into each other's drawers. I thought this meant that I had learned about love.

And then my artery tore. Caroline Myss's tape on love made me reconsider the physical event of my heart attack in the context of giving and forgiving. Perhaps I *was* here to learn about love.

To heal body and soul, I needed to learn more about how to actively forgive hurt from people who withhold love, how to resist the impulse to fill silences or make up for other people's stinginess. Recognition of the moment in which I began to feel hurt would be key. But how was I to do that? Ignoring hurt and muscling through was all I had known since I was thirteen. I had believed that if only I worked harder, were nicer, more generous, then my mother would live in spirit. That bad situations would improve by my effort alone. My overwhelming sense of responsibility had its good side, fanning an optimism like that of the White Queen in *Through the Looking Glass*, who told Alice, "Why sometimes I've believed as many as six impossible things before breakfast." The other side, which caused me to ignore my true feelings, was obviously not good for my health.

Even more important, I needed to follow the advice of the emperor Hadrian, as imagined by Marguerite Yourcenar: "Our great mistake is to try to exact from each person virtues which he does not possess, and to neglect the cultivation of those he has." I needed to learn how to see that though the cashier is sullen, she makes perfect change and that is enough.

42

HAVING SOLD OUR APARTMENT IN JANUARY, we needed a place to stay when Jack was working in Boston and I was in town for doctors. After entreating us to stay with her and Mark to no avail, Juliana had an idea.

"A club!" she said with triumph. "You could join the Harvard Club!"

I looked at her as though she had just suggested I dye my hair green.

Jack and I are decidedly not club people. We don't even own golf clubs. Clubs have always seemed to us to be exclusive societies of people who are too much alike, competitive places replicating the corporate world. Clubs were places that threw you out if you didn't follow rules that made no sense whatsoever, as happened to Jack at a dance when he took off his jacket and put it over the chilled shoulders of his pregnant first wife. My father came of age when "Catholics need not apply" for club membership, even terrific golfers. So while I had gone to graduate school at Harvard, becoming a member of its club was another thing altogether. It was tantamount to becoming an Episcopalian.

We joined the Harvard Club in desperation and were immediately ashamed of our preconceptions. World citizens of all colors and creeds sped through the foyer on their way to the squash courts. The staff was welcoming and solicitous. They even kept tabs on my whereabouts, noting my nap times, routing Jack's calls to the library or my room as though we were family. I was safe there.

At first I rarely ventured from the club without Jack or Juliana, but eventually its convenient location in Boston's Back Bay was too tempting. It was easy to walk out the door and embark on a short stroll along Commonwealth Avenue or Newbury Street, testing my independence one block at a time. Cabs were plentiful if I grew tired. (Taking the subway or a bus was out of the question; I kept imagining *what if it happens again and I can't get out.*)

It was all new, this city in which I had lived for almost twenty years. It was a startling place of continuous motion and cacophonous noise, so stimulating that I felt raw after just a few minutes of exposure to the throng. I had not felt its complexity and energy before. It terrified me.

I am in the day spa I discovered around the corner from the Harvard Club, waiting for a therapeutic massage, drinking lemon water, and looking at fashion magazines to discover how unfashionable I am.

A small woman with paintbrushes in her hands approaches me. "Would you like a makeover?"

Naturally, I am insulted. *What's so wrong with the way I look?* Besides, there is nothing I hate more than wearing makeup in the first place. And I certainly do not believe in making oneself over. It's like "starting over"—a complete lie and a waste of good experience.

I politely refuse her services, explaining that I am waiting for a massage, hoping that the awkward moment of finding myself wanting in her professional eyes is past. Then she sees my chest scar peeking through the terry-cloth wrap like the high Sierra and delicately inquires about it. I briefly share my story, hoping it will scare her away, but she is agitated in a most caring and concerned way.

"You must read *The Tibetan Book of Living and Dying* by Sogyal Rinpoche," she entreats.

I take mild offense again. It's taken a heck of a lot of effort to crawl out of the grave and into this spa, and I have no intention of dying. But her eyes are kind and urgent and I think, *Listen, pay attention, open like the dam at the end of the lake to let the winter melt flow.* She writes down the title and author, and when I leave I go immediately to a nearby bookstore and buy the book.

At first I read only the first few chapters; as with yoga, I felt it would be best to spend a long time in the beginner's class. And my first lesson from Tibetan Buddhism reverberated: experiences and people are not random but are meant to teach us something for use in this life or the next. My encounter with the makeup lady reinforced this lesson: a teacher had appeared bearing blush and guidance, just when I needed her. Had I not been paying attention, I would have dismissed the advice of a stranger, a woman who paints faces for a living, the archetypal messenger. When I returned to the spa a few weeks later, she had resigned and taken a new job. No one knew where she had gone.

The Buddhist notion of afterlife—that our spirits return again and again to this earth in different bodies, each time to learn new things—was not so far removed from Catholic visions of heaven. But even as a child I had never liked the sound of heaven as a final destination. It seemed, like a makeover, a waste of good experience. As the comedian George Carlin famously said, "After I've finally learned what life is about, it's all over." Instead of donning wings and hanging out with all the other good people up in the clouds, I always thought we should be doing something constructive with what we had learned during our time on earth. I prefer to believe in "old souls." We have all met or learned of people with wisdom beyond their years, from my nephew Chris, to our carpenter-friend, Bob, to Gandhi. I like to think that these wise people are old souls, reincarnate in a new body, bringing us the gift of their experiences from when time first began.

Like Caroline Myss, Sogyal Rinpoche suggested that my mysterious "cardiac event" was a chapter in my lifelong study of love. I was beginning to believe that even the psychic may have been on to something. Perhaps I was blessed with survival in order to learn something important about love, for this life and the next.

The idea that every person and event are here to teach us something also appealed to my practical side; here was a new trick I could employ when I sensed betrayal or the withholding of love! Instead of reacting, I could stop the energy drain that Dr. Myss described. Inquisitive by nature, I could *wonder* about the lesson a hurt offered and thereby detach emotionally and even forgive while remaining engaged. It was the difference between reacting and responding. It would take discipline and practice.

The foyer of Massachusetts Eye and Ear Medical Center seems even more bustling than around the corner at Mass General. I am here to see a throat specialist about my peculiar breathing, my first solo doctor's appointment. I am still congested and seem to breathe in short hesitations rather than deep, smooth inhalations. Could I have sustained damage to my throat from the intubation?

I walk toward a woman standing by the information desk who is carrying a clipboard and wearing an eager smile. She ushers me into a small booth, where I stand, in spite of the chair, waiting for someone to appear. *What is wrong with my throat? Is there a hole in it? Will I have to be operated on again?* Now that I'm here, come to think of it, I'm not so sure that I want to know what else is wrong with this body of mine. To calm myself, I practice focusing on my breath, but there is that hesitation whenever I inhale. The people around me wear the double mask of hope and despair found on all civilians wandering hospital corridors.

I am aware of stirrings and turn to face a woman who is not looking at me. She waves her hand in what seems to be a gesture, but her other hand is putting a sandwich in her mouth and maybe I'm mistaken. I hesitate.

"Excuse me?" I ask politely.

She points to the chair and turns her back, eating her sandwich. As I slide into the seat, I begin to unravel. It only takes a second. *How can you be rude to someone who is not well, who feels scared and vulnerable? If Jack were here . . .* But he is not, and I become hurt and angry. Then I catch myself. *This is how I react to thoughtless people.* I would never treat a patient, a customer, a person like this. But this woman is different from me, and now I have a choice of how to deal with it.

What is this woman here to teach me?

Immediately, my breathing becomes more natural and I feel my mind disconnect from my body and float a few steps back. The woman brusquely asks me questions, continuing to avoid my eyes and eat her sandwich. I answer directly, wondering about her life and the lesson she offers. There is a warm bath in my chest as the tension recedes.

Then, as the woman bends over the registration form to proof it, her face turned away from me at an angle, I notice a slight cleft palate which she is hiding behind her sandwich. I've had my first conscious lesson in protecting myself from the hurt that others can wreak because they are hurt themselves. *Did the lesson have to be so obvious, though? I get it, I get it.*

But I also think someone should give the woman better training.

In the throat specialist's waiting room, I am aware that I am being stared at by the staff—shy, furtive, respectful glances. A nurse brings me into an examination room and asks, "So, are you in the theater? Broadway?"

I look at him as though he is nuts. Then I see the photographs at the central desk, row after row of signed pictures from famous somebodies whose throats are their livelihoods. It hadn't occurred to me that this would be a big part of any throat specialist's practice.

"No, no," I stumble. "I'm nobody famous. Is that why people are staring at me?"

"Yes. You have such stage presence that we were taking bets on which of the performing arts was yours. We knew you weren't an opera singer; you're too thin."

Stage presence. I like that. It bucks me up a little. Here I am, still unable to stand with my shoulders back and they can't tell the difference. *Stage presence.*

When did a child's terror turn into performance? When did practice become stage presence? How will I ever know when I am turning it on? Can I turn it off? My stage presence has brought me friends, fun, jobs, adventure, and gotten me through some pretty challenging situations. If I step out of my accustomed role, what will I find? Who would I have been if the eyes of the world hadn't watched me lead my sisters and brother down the aisle toward our mother's casket, pretending to be Jackie Kennedy?

My trance is broken by the bustling entrance of the doctor I've seen racing between doors like the Roadrunner cartoon character. It's hard not to laugh at him when he slows down and comes into focus. He anesthetizes my throat and gently lowers a tiny camera on a long lead, easing it almost to my lungs. My gagging sounds metallic, like a garbage disposal eating a penny.

"Almost done. Keep breathing. Relax."

I am in a panic, drowning. I can't last much longer than this. I want to rip his hand away. And suddenly he is pulling the camera out and showing me the film of my throat. Nice and clear, although it looks rather like the interior of some sci-fi mollusk.

"What did you find?" I croak.

"Nothing," he replies, still looking at the screen. "You're remarkably clear for the speed with which those folks jammed the tube in. They did a great job at Mount Auburn Hospital."

"Nothing? Then what is blocking my breathing?" I ask, my voice normal, low and clear.

He turns to me. "Did you just hear that?"

"What?"

"Your voice was barely audible when I pulled out the tube. When I told you I found nothing, your voice returned to normal. What's wrong is muscle memory. Your throat remembers being traumatized and it is still spasming. It will go away."

I nearly break into song.

Emboldened by my solo mission to see the doctor, I decide to push the envelope and walk to Juliana's office on Newbury Street to surprise her for lunch. If I call her first, she will insist that I take a cab. She knows that for me, walking amid noise, traffic, and other people is like bushwhacking in a jungle. No, I cannot alarm Juliana. So I will sneak up on her.

I walk gingerly along Charles Street beneath gas lamps flickering in broad daylight, tippily weaving my way through window-shoppers as in a dream. Oh boldness! I venture into a few antique shops and talk to strangers, squandering a little energy and feeling it. In Marika's— the only antique shop with the atmosphere and prices of a country barn—I notice some oversized ivory-handled knives, five in one set, seven in another. Jack and I once bought twelve 1920s silver-plated spoons and forks at a flea market in Paris. We've paired them with our stainless-steel knives for years, not caring. Nothing matches in our lives and we like it that way. Sipping hot soup out of those huge spoons is the important thing: one slurp and it is Paris on a rainy day in a tiny restaurant near the Place des Vosges. I buy the knives—cheap, mismatched, and perfect.

Then I realize: I can't lift these, let alone carry them.

I panic, not wanting to tell strangers that I am incapable of carrying that small bag to Juliana's, that I am afraid I will die of exertion along the way. Then I ask them to hold the knives for a day so that I can bring my husband by for the final decision, something I've never done. It feels quaint.

I enter the Public Gardens, past children sitting on the bronze ducklings with mothers fluttering protectively around them and snapping pictures. Looking at the serpentine paths ahead of me in this graceful, frozen garden, I see a war zone. I didn't anticipate the dizzy feeling of exposure in this open space, surrounded by strangers who won't know what to do if the box fires or if I fade from exhaustion. Every sound, every sight has equal importance and I am filling up with chaos.

Beep. Beep. Beep.

Is that the box?

I stop and listen to my body, my mind a jumble. I walk carefully to a bench and sit down, ready for the hit, cursing my bravado, holding my cell phone for dear life.

Nothing. But I think I'll sit here awhile longer to be sure . . .

Then I hear the beeping sound again. It is a truck backing up on Beacon Street warning everyone to get out of its way. I am safe on my bench. I need to read my booklet on the ICD again. Does it make any sound before the horse kicks me in the chest?

Several blocks down Newbury Street, I fall on the button for Juliana's elevator as though it is a fire alarm. The elevator shakes and rattles me up to her sunny office crammed with paintings. She is glad to see me but also stern as we walk across the street to lunch. With the delivery of breadsticks to the table, she relaxes and we giggle wickedly about my triumph as though I'd sneaked a peak at the nuns' underwear on the line behind school. Then Juliana insists on driving me to Marika's to pick up the knives and back to the Harvard Club. Great idea! I won't have to tell Jack a thing. The knives will just suddenly appear at dinner.

43

WINTER GAVE ITS FINAL PUSH and the lake moaned at night as temperatures dipped and the ice expanded. Sometimes it cracked violently like a whip. Sometimes it sounded like a woman softly laughing far away. Sometimes it raced like a lit fuse to crash with a *whump* into our point, shaking the entire house. The night music of the shifting ice was as companionable as the loons in summer fog.

Under the glow of my reading light, I had progressed a few more pages in *The Tibetan Book of Living and Dying* when I came upon another astonishing thought: the moment we are conceived is the moment we start dying. Come to think of it, Bob Dylan sang about this in "It's All Right, Ma." Why hadn't I considered it before? Suddenly I had lots of company. We were all dying as we lived.

My year of recovery with its infinitesimal adjustments had brought me face-to-face with what I now learned was the Buddhist concept of impermanence. There is only one law in the universe that never changes: all things change and all things are impermanent, even death, because we do not know when and how death will occur or what happens afterward. In its own mutability, death is the apotheosis of all change, which is why it is the most difficult shared human experience. Beginning at birth, practice adjusting to life's changes and betrayals prepares us for how we will handle the big one.

"It is only when we believe things to be permanent that we shut off the possibility of learning from change," wrote Sogyal Rinpoche. "If we shut off this possibility, we become closed, and we become grasping. Grasping is the source of all our problems. Since impermanence to us spells anguish, we grasp onto things desperately, even though all things change. We are terrified of letting go, terrified, in fact, of living at all, since *learning to live is learning to let go*." [italics mine]

As I put down the book, I considered my primal, swift self-assessment when death came for me in the emergency room of Mount Auburn Hospital: I was content with the sudden change in my plans and prepared to go. I had kept such thoughts to myself because they would have been alarming to others. But it was true. In that split-second review, I knew my life had been good. I'd done my best. I was at peace. There was no terror in the moment. In saying as much to the bearded doctor I'd imagined bending over me, perhaps I was actually speaking to God. In my acceptance, I bent and survived, like the birch trees of our ice storm. I saw the faces of all the people who had been caring for me since May 12. They, too, had yielded to change, and in so doing steered me and consequently themselves back into this world with love.

I turned out the light and went to bed. Enough for one day. Before

I closed my eyes, though, I checked to see if the light at the end of the lake was on, my companion in the black expanse.

Was it my heightened sensitivity, or had there been a flood of new reports on cardiovascular disease? I cut out every article and read all the relevant newsletters and books. Unfortunately, the studies were not usually encouraging for a young woman who wanted to live more than ten years. One study announced that—good news!—women will survive as long as men postoperatively, whereas they were previously believed to have a higher mortality rate. Then the Spanish announced that women have more severe cardiac events than men and are more likely to die in the first year afterward. Then an American study corrected that by factoring in that women who have heart attacks generally have them when they are much older than men, in their seventies, which is why they don't live long.

Whew.

Over time I began to see that the study of cardiovascular disease was another example of impermanence. Being the number-one American killer, it was in the news every week with new information of some kind. Findings both reinforced and contradicted each other. Breakthroughs occurred, only to be superseded by new breakthroughs. I learned to read with detachment—eventually becoming grateful that I had a disease that received so much research attention. I called Marc less often, saving what I couldn't make sense of in my little notebook for our next meeting.

Gracie the parrot is on my mind today as I look out the kitchen window toward a snow-blanketed Mount Washington. Even if predators hadn't found her right away, she must be long dead by now, frozen. And here I am all warm and cozy in my home on a lake in western Maine, resting in the dead of winter. Everything is hushed, with only the occasional buzz of a snowmobile across the lake. Icicles drip in the blazing sun, forming troughs around the house.

Good thing the ice is covered with snow, so skating cannot tempt me today. Skating is forbidden to me now—a fall and a blow to the head too risky with the blood thinners. I'm thinking about buying a helmet and it makes me sad, probably the way motorcyclists felt when riding without a helmet became illegal.

Then the itching under my skin comes to the surface and I know just what I need to do. I'm breaking out. The lake itself poses no risk; ice fishing shacks and trucks have been on it for weeks. But fear of an arrhythmia is my constant companion. First, I call Jack. I have not lost my head so much that I will venture forth without telling him. He protests a little but knows it is pointless. I strap on my athletic heart monitor to be sure that I don't overexert myself. (Exercising in the cold puts more pressure on the heart, so the rate tends to increase faster than in warm weather.) Dressing for my adventure, I layer my clothes as I was taught in rehab so I can zip and unzip as needed. My pack holds a cell phone, tissues, and a water bottle. Then I stride through my snow-covered garden and onto the open lake, now a sparkling white field. The sun is high, sky clear and perfect with cold. There's a dusting of fresh snow cleaner than clouds, blue shadows streaking it. I am squinting, even with sunglasses.

This is not a day to be wasted inside.

I set out on snowmobile tracks for Rob's Village, a cluster of colorful, patched-together ice houses that a neighbor moves to the middle of the lake every year. He's always got a box of wine and food there for viewing the annual Musher's Bowl, the Maine state dogsled races, which pass by our house to the other end of the lake and back. As I walk on the crusted tracks, I look down and enjoy my aerial view. The world at my feet looks like the three-dimensional topographical map of Jack's beloved Denali at the Boston Museum of Science. The tracks are my map and this is my mountain, though there will be no increase in altitude today.

When I look up again, the expanse of lake and sky and my freedom overwhelm me, giving me vertigo. This is not Boston's Public Gardens; there is no bench to catch me. Then I think of Gracie flying recklessly, high and free above the dun-colored field.

I know why she did it.

I know why she soared, as giddy as I feel from the sting of cold, fresh air in my nostrils. On this dazzling, frigid day—just weeks before the lake begins its slow melt and boats once again float freely—impatience nudges my terror out of the way. *If this is incautious, then I don't care.* Today, at last, I am not afraid to be completely alone in wide, open space. It has taken almost ten months to get to this point—just as Stan, Torch's PA, had said it would when he held my shaking hand after the box fired twice in the gray morning light of Ellison-8.

I am beginning to trust the ice beneath my feet. I am beginning to believe that my body will not fail me. Tiny cyclones of powder twirl in the distance, and I am happier than I've been in ages. This busting out is not an irresponsible act of rebellion. It is as sensible as kicking through the drugs when the doctors wanted me to be still.

Newly confident about my returning physical strength, I switched to an Iyengar yoga class, like the one I'd taken in Cambridge. I missed Zoe. We'd spoken a few times by phone, but it didn't compare to the privilege of being in her class. An athletic and precise form of yoga concentrating on alignment, Iyengar was permitted, Marc said, only if I breathed comfortably through my nose and avoided advanced inversions (like I even *wanted* to do a head-stand!). If I started to breathe through my mouth, a sign of strain, I was to come out of any pose. My new teacher, Scott, explained that this was how Iyengar yoga should be done anyway, in tune with the breath.

Yoga is Sanskrit for binding, joining, wholeness. Its purpose is to raise consciousness, thereby uniting body and spirit. The physical practice of yoga leads the way to greater spiritual awareness as the body first absorbs its teachings so that your mind can use them. For example, when you become more conscious of a muscle in a pose, you can soften it, release its tension. In letting go, in being flexible, you discover its strength. Just as in life.

In resuming my yoga practice, I brought so much more understanding to it than before the heart attack. I was tentative and sore, but I was there on my skid-resistant yoga mat, feet firmly planted on the earth. Soon my shoulders softened and lay back a bit, giving up their load. I began to gain a little muscle weight and could hold my own in the north wind a bit better. As winter days grew longer and the edges of the lake grew squishy, my body became lighter and more malleable, on a parallel healing track with my mind.

By winter's end, in addition to yoga, I had three practices to help me be in life again. I practiced harnessing intuition, our most powerful energetic force. I tried to halt energy drains from hurt by immediately asking myself what I could learn from the situation. And I practiced accepting impermanence by continuing to observe nature, learning to look at life's many betrayals as change, the same stuff that makes daffodils appear like surprises every spring.

Mind you, none of these ideas were new to me. Wise people had tried to get them through my thick skull through fairy tales, literature, poetry, history, conversation, and example. But it took illness to bring them home with clarity and urgency. I no longer had anything to lose and I had everything to gain; that allowed me finally to absorb what I needed to learn. As Caroline Myss wrote, "Truth is no more than a prayer away at all times. The only thing that blocks it—if you looked and asked yourself clearly—is that you are so terrified of how truth can change your life."

SECOND SPRING

44

In early March, Jack gave a speech at the Museum of Science to introduce a special showing of the new IMAX film, *Everest*. He spoke well and movingly, stirring the crowd with tales of trust, commitment, teamwork, adventure, loss, and reward played out in thin air. Jack had always believed that mountains were metaphors. His climbing experience had been superb training for this past year. As he spoke to the rapt crowd, he told me later, he was also seeing himself in a dimly lit hospital room with machines blinking and beeping; he was seeing himself supervising my walking-training on Beacon Hill; he was seeing himself purchasing and testing the equipment that would ensure my safety and his peace of mind when he left me in Maine; he was seeing us enduring the separations and surviving our sea-level ice storm. We were as tight a team as anyone on Everest. He had me on his rope.

When he was done, Jack bowed slightly with pleasure and relief, sneaking me a vulnerable look. I smiled and he stood up straight, sparkling. Then we went into the Omni theater and I walked slowly up the steep stairs to our seats at the top, eschewing the elevator. It was my first mountain since our annual winter climb of Mount Washington just three months before my heart attack. I edged my way along the row of seats to Dr. Rich Moscicki, who had conspired to save my life the minute he saw Jack's tail-lights receding down Commonwealth Avenue. Rich applauded quietly. I tried to breathe normally to deserve his happiness, to hide how exhausted I really was with a smile as wide as the screen. My mind was young, but my body felt old.

"Are you all right?" Rich asked, concerned.

"Yeah, I just need a minute to catch my breath."

Maybe, just maybe, I thought, I could walk partway up Mount Washington with Jack and his kids next February.

Dad has just returned home from a follow-up appointment for a cataract operation. My sister Leesa has moved in with him to be his nurse and companion during a break from work. After two weeks, Leesa will bring Dad to Callie's house, where he will stay until he feels confident enough to live on his own again. My nephew Chris is looking forward to watching ball games with his grandfather, exchanging comments with sportscasters' authority.

I am frustrated that I can't help in some way, even though I am the one who is no longer working. After all, Dad and I are on the same sleeping schedules and have to eat the same diet. No, no, no, they say. You and Dad together? He couldn't survive the anxiety over you. What if the box fired? Besides, Marc says you're not supposed to drive yet. I know they are right, but it rankles. I try to make up for it by sending frozen chicken soup by overnight mail.

My phone call catches Dad alone in his kitchen, making tea while Leesa is off on errands.

"Deb, I've always been alone," Dad says. His tone of voice suggests that I am arguing the point. "I *like* being alone."

"I know, Dad . . ."

"But I can't be alone now. This eye thing. It's rocked me. I can't drive; I can't do things for myself. My balance is off; getting in and out of the tub is . . . It's my loss of independence that's got me thinking. This is what it's like . . . when I can't be alone."

He cannot say the real words. I cannot hear them either. He has always been strong as a bull. Now old age has dropped on him like a garage door. It took only eighty-five brief years. I am aware that it came on fast after I got sick, but I push this thought aside quickly, like brambles.

I reflect on my own jump in age, and think that maybe Dad won't feel so frustrated if he knows I'm frustrated, too. I remind him that I have not driven farther than the bank in almost a year. He is shocked.

"A year? How can that be, Deb?"

I explain the box again. He is silent.

I also tell him that I had one of my "moments" yesterday when my spanking-new, neon-purple, high-tech life vest arrived. Keenly anticipating the coming summer, I'd ordered it from a nautical supply store in Portland harbor. It is a slim one that windsurfers use, cut wide in the armpits and perfect for me; it won't rub creepily against the box. Marc has given me permission to swim if I use this, after I confessed that my husband is not a suitable swimming guardian. (Once a certified Junior Maine Guide, Jack knows no stroke but the crawl and can do that only with his head in the water, swimming with no direction whatsoever. His stroke is dazzlingly beautiful as long as it lasts.)

I tell Dad that I had felt so clever when I thought of the life-vest solution. That I had imagined showing it off to my nurse, Debbie, when she visits this summer. How happily I pulled it out of its cardboard box, unwrapped the tissue paper, and tried it on. Then I began to cry torrents, all alone in the kitchen. To be blessed with living on the water and yet prevented from swimming with long strokes from our point to the next! To be forbidden to swim naked under the moon with the bats swooping in hot, steamy blackness. I tell Dad that I cried for the loss of freedom and spontaneity that only the confined can truly understand—and I was hardly confined compared to many citizens of my new world.

I can tell that Dad is thinking deeply about this. Then he makes a confession of his own: sometimes at night he pees sitting down—it's simply easier when he is so unsteady. We laugh. I consider confessing that Jack does, too, when he knows he's too groggy. But then I don't. Dad could think I haven't understood what he is really saying.

I cannot insult him by saying that I completely understand. Fear—of falling on the ice and setting the box off or inducing a hematoma, of walking across the street and not having the adrenaline push I once had to flee a careless driver—has given me a taste of old age. But I respect the difference between my chronological place and Dad's, and regret that I cannot truly go the distance to keep my father company in his new world. Death has crawled into bed with Jack and me, but I still have age on my side. What Dad and I have in common is our greediness for life, born of our new limitations. Sometimes we may seem impatient.

But this much I do know: it's beginning to drive me crazy not to be able to jump in my car and just go, go anywhere. Before this moment I was too afraid. Now I want my wheels back.

They told me to get there early to avoid standing in line. I am no longer any good at standing in line, both by temperament and strength. It's a cold, drizzly, spring morning in Maine following a night of wet snow that fell with messy plops. I open the heavy door to the basement of the Town Hall with difficulty, easing it open a crack, shoving my toe in to wedge it farther open, then inserting my shoulder until I create a space just wide enough to slide through sideways. The representative from the Department of Motor Vehicles won't be here until ten and I am pleased to be forty-five minutes early.

There are already twenty people in the room ahead of me. In Maine, we like to get places early, just in case.

My companions are all much older than me and staring with curiosity at the young woman who can't even open a door. I want to explain what Torch told me about my chest and exertion, about why I am not as robust as they are, though I wear a youthful disguise. But their stares hold no judgment. I am merely a diversion. I pull a folding metal chair up to a cafeteria table and wait like the rest.

It is a room full of caps—baseball caps of all kinds and colors, some with the logos of local businesses. Some of them are made of mesh, worn even on this wet, bone-chilling spring day, on any day year-round. In Maine men's caps seem welded to their bodies. I often wonder if they sleep in them. Do they put their caps on as soon as they get out of bed, like a prosthesis or dentures? Do they wear them in the shower?

The atmosphere in the freshly painted basement is festive. The men joke with one another. They are hardworking men whose daily lives are rituals, interrupted occasionally by the outside world for things like renewing licenses. Two elderly women sit close together in a corner so they can catch up on things. I am shy. They can probably tell I am a Flatlander. Lil once told me that I am the only Flatlander she has ever liked. She's about to become a Flatlander herself; she told me that God told her to move to Maryland.

An efficient young woman in slacks and a matching sweater arrives with boxes and begins to set up shop at the front of the room. She represents the state and will decide if we are worthy of driving or not. In one of the boxes is a device that will assist her: an eye-testing machine.

"Who's first?"

One by one we file respectfully to the desk as though we are approaching the altar for Communion. The men's hats come off only long enough to peer into the eye-testing machine. The rest of us can hear her questions and people's mumbled answers. The first woman waits for her friend to be finished and they walk out together, still talking. I am beginning to sweat. I have heard very clearly that one of the questions is "Has anything changed in your health?" Then more to the point, "Do you have a heart condition?"

Wow, I'll say!

I am in a panic. This is not a multiple-choice question. One by one these people who shuffle up to the desk, who take a long time with the eye test, who can barely hear the questions, are being given licenses. It seems that every time I have built myself up—adjusting my expectations, recalibrating, finding happiness in my corral—I meet another situation where I am reminded that I must prematurely navigate the world of the elderly. In this country, a car is life itself, freedom, self-determination. If you can't drive, you are isolated, forgotten, vulnerable. Old. I wish things were different, wish we would install a better public transportation system. But America loves cars.

Sweating on my cold metal chair as my turn draws closer and closer, I am in a moral quandary. What is the responsible way for me to answer this question? When does embracing impermanence become caving in, giving up, the abnegation of spirit?

It is the next man's turn. He is huge and has to try three times before he is up on his feet, swaying with his son to steady him. They finally make it to the desk and we all want to cheer. The official is respectful. She patiently waits for him to sit down again, then slowly takes him through every test. He fails. She tells him that if he returns with a note from his doctor, he can try again. She says it nicely, with no pity—as though this is a small misunderstanding, as though there is a chance still. But we all feel his despair and embarrassment. He's been given his death sentence. He will never drive again. The official runs through the entire process with another supplicant before the old gentleman even makes it to the door.

It's my turn. I fly through the eye test. She gives me a look implying, "I know this is a bother for you, just a formality." She is more collegial with me, lighter.

Then she asks offhandedly, "Has anything changed in your health?"

I am a Girl Scout. I have never been able to lie.

"Yes."

She looks up at me, surprised. And then I race to the close.

"I have a heart condition."

She speaks quickly, unnerved.

"Has your doctor got you on any medications? If so, I need a note from him before I can give you a license."

Unwittingly, she has revealed the game. And then I think of what Dad would do. My life is at stake. So I lie.

"I'm not on any medications."

I am red with heat and trying my hardest to look casual. Focusing on my breathing. Thank heavens for yoga.

She smiles with obvious relief. "Well, then, everything is fine. If you were on medications, we couldn't proceed without your doctor's permission." (Since then, Marc has approved.)

"I guess I'm overreacting a little," I say, warming to my role. "I just had my annual checkup and they discovered a slight mitral valve prolapse. They say it's nothing, but I'm still adjusting. I've never had anything wrong before. I guess you wouldn't count that as a heart problem." A little giggle, just for emphasis.

"Nah. I have it too. It's nothing. Did they tell you about taking penicillin when you have your teeth cleaned?"

"Yes. I hope I remember to. It'll be the first time I've ever taken anything stronger than aspirin."

We laugh together. I try not to grab the license and run.

45

In Boston that April for my quarterly checkup with Marc, we met the man I'd been tracking since Jack giggled in my rehab class on drugs. Dr. Ned Cassem was not only a psychiatrist, but also a Jesuit priest and the hospital chaplain, which I knew would be a comfort to Jack, whose childhood Sunday dinners had been packed with lively priests. The priests had been his father figures when his own father let him down, drunkenly raving at the head of the table with young Jack next to him, feeling responsible and ashamed.

For a long time I didn't tell Jack I had scheduled him for therapy; he had continually rebuffed my overtures. Finally I sprang the first appointment on him when we were out for a walk. He protested, but only a little. It was time. Jack had needed to thrash around on his own for a while before he was ready. We decided that I would join them for fifteen minutes of Jack's first session. When Ned bustled in, glowing from within like an apricot, Jack visibly relaxed. The timing was right and we had found a holy man to help Jack become whole. In fact, the root of "holy" in Old English is *haelan*, to heal, and in Indo-European languages it is from *kailo*, meaning whole or uninjured.

In just a few sessions, Ned took Jack deep into his past and uncovered the terror that was paralyzing him, causing him to believe that every breath was my last, to panic if I did not answer the phone in three rings. It stemmed from his childhood experience with Dylan Thomas's "first death"—the fear that his mother would die when his father was drunk. When I was in the hospital, hovering between this life and the next, he had returned to the nightmare of his childhood, to the threat of being completely alone. Ned created a safe atmosphere in which Jack could remember his father—so kind and funny when he wasn't drunk—chasing his mother with lamps or vases, while Jack held his twin sister's hand and prayed to the statue of the Blessed Virgin Mother in the living room, prayed that Mom would not die that night. As he said the words again, he realized that this was the same prayer he had chanted watching a clock tick at MGH while doctors assaulted my body to save my life. When Jack emerged from his final session with this insight, he floated beside me as we walked down the street. His first love had not died, and neither had I.

Still, Jack will never be totally relaxed with me. But understanding his reaction helps him to manage it and helps us to talk about it.

In his vigilance, Jack never chafed, as many caregivers would, at the skeleton clinging to him on the way to the toilet. In fact, he was delighted with my dependence on him; my husband needs to be totally trusted the way some men need money or sex. Ever since he was a child unable to save his mother from his father's alcoholism, or his father from himself, he had dreamed of responsibility. By holding my hand and guiding me through life, Jack also protects himself because at his side is someone who loves him completely, without violence or changeability.

Occasionally I try to throw off his hovering and am cranky. Only occasionally. The truth is that my need for him and the protection he guarantees has made me more independent than ever in *spirit* because my guardian does not censor me. I am more free in my corral with Jack than I ever was on a business trip to Dallas.

During my quarterly checkup with Marc, we broached the idea of traveling to Bermuda in a couple of weeks. After all, my box readings indicated no arrhythmias in the last few months, and I was still stable. Our bold talismans were the tickets I had already bought with my expiring frequent-flyer miles. Positive thinking had gotten us this far in our journey—why not to Bermuda?

We chose Bermuda for our big adventure because it had been a haven for my family after my mother's death. When we were in our late teens and twenties, Dad began a tradition that lasted ten years: we spent Christmas in Bermuda, descending on that civilized island like chattering magpies. December in Bermuda suited us; we didn't mind the cloudy weather because our pale skin couldn't handle much sun and the rates were cheap. All seven of us, plus in-laws, crowded into two apartments on South Road near Horseshoe Bay and sped away from each other on mopeds when we needed privacy. It would do me good to return to a place of fond memories where I knew every bend in the road.

Marc approved the adventure quickly, throwing us off-balance. Smiling mischievously, he explained that I would be in good hands in Bermuda if anything went wrong; he knew the local doctors well, he said. *Knew the doctors well?*

"Bermuda is a big heart donor location."

We looked puzzled.

"You know, with all the moped accidents."

While stunning and true, it was also Marc's first attempt at humor since we had known him. We looked at it as another test that my body had passed.

Speaking of which, my body needed new clothes. All fall and winter I had given away clothing that no longer fit and I would no longer wear. It was an interesting process no less profound than asking, "Who am I?" I had taken my time with decisions about what went and what I kept. From the very beginning it was a liberating experience. *Anybody want this gray suit? How about a nice navy wool dress shapely as a sack?*

The clothes brought good memories, too. One suit reminded me of a day I spent working with engineers in the plant of a major automobile parts manufacturer, covered with a smock, grease booties on my Cinderella pumps, large goggles wrapped around my face. I loved working with engineers on documentation; their minds were always interesting. The good people I had met as I crisscrossed the country would always be in my life, in memories or in person. My perfect suits never mattered to them anyhow. In purging my closet I was purging the other experiences which had taken my soul off course.

While always slender, I was now built like a hipless teenager—causing wide eyes from my sisters, the envy of friends, and a catalog shopping spree. The craze for stretch fabrics was at its height and I had no bumps on my body left to hide. I bought a few slimmer, more fashionable items that I could never have worn in business, making me feel light as a prancing runway model. Packing for Bermuda was like opening birthday packages: I assembled my new spring outfits in a tizzy of combinations. For the plane ride, I donned some skinny capri pants that made Jack roll his eyes; it was still thirty degrees in Maine.

With the car running, Jack went into the house one more time and discovered I'd left my huge straw hat *again* on the bench. With a final

"Do you have your drugs? Your vitamins? Your sunscreen? All the medical phone numbers?" he locked the door on this long, last year and released the brake. Tame as Bermuda was, we felt positively reckless with anticipation.

As we crossed our dirt causeway, we discovered that the deep frozen ruts of winter were becoming soft like rubber. The air was steamy with evaporating snow. The mourning doves, always the first birds we notice in spring, fluttered off the driveway and into the trees. Maine was flirting with its annual thaw, which would struggle along for a few weeks.

We call it Mud Season—an unpredictable, in-between season with a life of its own, sinking us in mud and thrilling us with the smell of earth that has been buried under snow for five months. We love it for its promise. We dread it for the reality, which makes driving down a long dirt road with a car full of groceries a pioneer's adventure. We are happiest when it begins and when it is over.

It looked like the timing of our trip to Bermuda was perfect: we'd be gone during the worst of it.

We have our game plan down. Jack will carry our luggage and I am not to lift a thing but my purse. I am to walk slowly behind him so he can scan the terminal for machines that would turn my box off, confusion that would drain me, and exact destinations so we don't waste energy walking in circles. He is an FBI agent ready to take the hit for me and proud of the role. I am feeling both foolish and grateful. Being in Logan Airport for the first time in a year is overwhelming. How did I live in this environment, flying to meetings all over North America week after week over the last fourteen years? It is a loud and alien place, a blaring, senseless television set. The air is stingy. People weave like sleepwalkers.

I perch on an abandoned luggage wagon while Jack attempts to get us upgraded. He gestures with his hands, touches his heart, and points at me as if he is mute. I smile nicely at the reservation attendant and then realize this is probably not what I should do, given my rosy cheeks. I should probably try to look pathetic. Or maybe I do look pathetic and I am kidding myself. For all Jack's fussing over me,

I know that he is right: this entire atmosphere is draining me. He is expert at anticipating energy drains, a skill that will challenge me for the rest of my life. On trips to the grocery store, I still automatically start to help the clerk bag groceries—until Jack gives me one of his looks. *Conserve energy, Deborah. Stand back from life a little.*

Success! We are whisked past the lines and sent to the gate to board as first class passengers. I slow as we approach the security checkpoint. It never appeared like an enemy fortress before. The wand and the security gate could turn off my box, maybe just at the moment I need it. I used to breeze through the gate, occasionally setting the alarms off with a piece of jewelry. Even in my rush I was never cross with the security guards; I was always grateful for their protection. Now I am tensing for battle. *What if someone forces me to go through the security door? What if someone aims a wand at me? How far away from this stuff is safe?* On the other side of the gate I see the man with the wand, passing it over and around a businessman. The wand looks as menacing to me as a billy club.

Jack to the rescue. He is gesturing again and a man points to a corner by the side of the gates. We obey and are greeted by a tiny female leprechaun with pretty bones and the wrinkled skin of a lifelong smoker. She twinkles up at silver-haired Jack, thinking he is the one with the ICD who needs to be frisked. He presents me instead.

"Oh, dear. Not you, dear. You're far too young. You have a defibrillator? I can't believe it. Tsk, tsk. But so thin! Oh, what a shame."

She fusses over me lovingly, giving me a mother's back rub more than a body search. I begin to tear. *Please don't say nice things to me, please, or I'll fall apart right here.* When she is done she hugs me. She comes up to my armpits and smells comfortingly of perfume and smoke like my Aunt Katherine.

"I'll pray for you, darlin'. I'll pray for you every day. You have a lovely time. Oh, dear."

Jack takes my arm. We've been blessed by a pint-size Saint Christopher, the patron of travelers.

Feeling the plane lift off the ground and away from Boston is as dramatic for me as being airlifted out of a war zone and heading home—home being freedom from fear, a peace of mind I once took for granted. Only a couple of months before, we thought I would never travel again. A few months before that, Jack had thought I might emerge brain-damaged from the anesthesia. Now here we are on an airplane headed for Bermuda's fragrant spring and its welcoming warm, soft air.

As Jack and I walked down the rattling aluminum stairs to the tarmac, the first gust of sweet air was like aromatherapy, filling me with hilarious memories of our family tumbling down the same stairs to the same tarmac years ago, Dad carrying our rapidly defrosting Christmas turkey in an old green book bag, leaking juices.

After dropping our bags at our small, old-fashioned hotel in Hamilton, we headed to the moped rental shop. While thrilled and astonished that Marc had given us permission to ride, I had misgivings about not driving my own bike. I had always loved the sensuality of swerving with the road, the independence of stopping and meandering at will, the wind in my face. To ride passively behind Jack would be another reminder of my complete dependence on him.

I also knew that Jack was a living horror on a moped. For an American dyslexic, the roads in any part of the United Kingdom are a nightmare because of the reversal of left and right. Jack was no exception. He was especially challenged by "roundabouts," often circling round and round about them, too afraid to get off. Now, for the first time in my life, I was to climb on the back of a moped with someone else driving—and the driver was Jack.

He was more terrified than I was, but he had to keep his eyes open.

The paperwork complete, we pushed off. I shut my eyes tight against all the stone walls we would hit, the hedges we would tear through, the curves we would miss to plunge into the ocean, never to be seen again.

Instead, we moved like one muscle. Of course.

Jack wobbled us into balance. I navigated, speaking instructions into his good ear, pointing instead of saying left and right. We purred along Front Street with sparkling shops on our left and the harbor on our right. We stopped and balanced at lights. We hit the first rotary and sailed through. He pulled on the handlebars and accelerated up the hill. We were free! White Easter lilies nodded in our jet stream as we passed, releasing their heady perfume. Hedges covered with purple and magenta bougainvillea watched over our giddy flight. We were the luckiest people in the world when we arrived at Horseshoe Bay, giggling, drunk with happiness.

And there was the ocean as it had always been, calmly pouring in and rumbling out, in, out, in, out, lingering just long enough to leave a damp scalloped edge on the sand.

46

WHEN DOES WINTER END and spring begin? When does sleep become wakefulness? When did I stop assuming that every beep on the street meant that my box had just switched off because of a giant magnet? When did fatigue come to mean a bad day and not a downward slide? When did I begin saving my reading on heart disease for my checkups with Marc instead of calling him daily with every bit of news, scared or hopeful that it applied to me? When exactly did my terror turn into attentiveness? Can you pinpoint the exact moment in which change occurs? Is it when you approach the door, when you pass through it, when you step out on the other side, or when you lock it behind you? Change is all of these, a blurring of before and after, a threshold with indistinct borders—like Mud Season.

I have always loved another threshold: the gloaming, that twilight moment between day and night that will not be held to a time on the clock. It was a word my maternal grandmother taught me as we sat in her garden of snapdragons and petunias, watching the light leave us. It is the pause when a brilliant sunset softens into indistinctness and calm. Our lake quiets in the gloaming and becomes still as the mountains in the distance. Reflecting back on my reaction to the tightening in my chest, I realized that I, too, had been as still as a quieting lake, pausing in the gloaming of my life.

Observing these natural transitions reminds me of observing one's breath in yoga—in, out, in, out, always noticing the *pause* between breaths, the space that the pause inhabits. Tibetan Buddhists call these pauses in life *bardos*. The greatest and most charged bardo is the moment of death, but bardos occur continuously throughout life. They are junctures when the possibility of liberation or enlightenment is heightened—like the moment you step toward the edge of a precipice for the view, or swerve up a muddy causeway on the way to the airport with your heart in your throat, or have a massive heart attack and stand at the edge of your life.

Somewhere in Mud Season, in the gloaming of winter, I began to live again—just as they had said I would, almost twelve months after a bomb exploded in my chest.

It was Ice Out the day we returned from Bermuda. Mainers consider it good luck to bear witness, and Lil declared that she'd seen it happen that morning as she hung sheets on our line for the wind to dry. She left her announcement in a note as though celebrating a birth.

Ice Out marks the end of Mud Season, and the true beginning of spring in Maine, even though the vernal equinox is usually past. The lake's melting process is long and slow, often beginning in late March, when ice fishermen know instinctively that they had better haul their huts off the lake or lose them for good. The snow-mobilers no longer buzz by. Quiet returns to the lake as it does in early fall when summer guests leave. No one goes for walks on the lake anymore. Puddles of water float on the ice like swimming pools on cruise ships. Then whole sections of ice disappear and open water sloshes through. As the winds off Mount Washington blow with April fury and churn up water eager to see the sun again, the ice is pushed in floes downstream to crash on our point, where it piles up like sheet metal in a junkyard. More huge floes sail by to the dam at Stevens Brook, opened full tilt to welcome the spring melt. One day, the last ice floe passes by like a homecoming queen. This is Ice Out. The precise day is usually in late April, but everyone in town will declare that it happened on a different day. It is a violent bardo with a peaceful resolution. Once again we sleep to the sound of water lapping rhythmically at our shore.

On cue a couple of weeks after Ice Out, Lucia pulled down the driveway in her orange Volkswagen bus filled with rakes and shovels; it was time to uncover the garden and see how everything had fared over the winter. I'd been anticipating her arrival for days with deep excitement, not knowing exactly when she would come. There is never a schedule for anything in Maine except school, and even that has exceptions. People try their hardest to show up or deliver the goods when they intend to, but it never happens. Whole days go by with no-shows and no explanatory phone calls, and suddenly huge trucks appear to dig a cesspool just as you are feeding dinner to hungry guests from the city who already think you are nuts to live in the middle of nowhere.

Lucia brought flats of pansies in colors I had never seen before and I potted them happily on the picnic table as her crew carefully lifted off mulch and dug holes. I loved this annual ritual. Jack had planted the first rhododendron the year we were engaged, awakening my genetic passion for dirty hands, passed on to me from my maternal grandmother and Dad's brother, Uncle Curt, whose Cape Cod garden grew like a tropical jungle.

When everything is uncertain in the rest of my life, I can always depend on the cycles of the garden. I know my routines of care for fragile roots and invasive plants. In the garden, there are known good guys, like ladybugs, and known bad guys, like aphids. There is the confidence that most things will grow if planted sensibly. And if you make a mistake, you can always dig it up. Our sour, windswept land slowly spoke to me over the years (gardeners talk like this, communing with their dirt like other people talk with their dogs), telling me where to sculpt a curving stone path, where to make it soft with pine needles, where a stone wall should go, which corner needed height and fat bushes, which needed perennials that could survive the snow dumped by the plow.

In the beginning, I made classic mistakes by insisting that I had sun in the garden, just as I had once clung stubbornly to my belief in Santa Claus long after I knew the truth. The sun does indeed pass through various corners of my garden; I can feel it occasionally on my back as I dig. But it took a few years before I accepted that it passes through like a train speeding between tunnels and discovered the more dependable joys of shade gardening. Some of my mistakes remain, all straggly in search of the blazing light they need and deserve for having tried to like it here for so long. Slowly I pull them out and trade them to Lucia for more appropriate and sturdy choices. Some of these don't like it here either. But I grant them a good long chance to prove their mettle before I give them up. I give them time, as the gods have given me.

So, my garden is in a constant state of movement. Impermanence. Lucia calls it my instinct for relentless reorganization. Some of this she approves of—it aerates the soil. In other cases, she begs me to stop, to let some corner grow in peace without my pestering it to be better than it is. Possibility has always been my weakness.

Watching Lucia's crew plunge shovels into hard, sandy soil and begin to dig a new bed filled me with deep satisfaction. Then it dawned on me. She had done this for me a year ago, seducing me with pansies when I'd come home to Maine for good and ached to do the work I had always taken such pleasure in. I looked at my arms, expecting to see the pale, thin things they were then. Now they had shape, sort of, and a Bermuda sunburn. I could almost stand straight now, too. I could stand while potting the flowers. I could last longer than fifteen minutes. It was spring and I was being resurrected like my garden, like the tree frogs in our swamp peep-peep-peeping to the world that they are *here*.

47

JACK AND I WENT TO BOSTON for the week of May 12, the first anniversary of my heart attack. Feeling skittish as the date approached, we had concluded that it would be a good idea to be with the friends and family who had been closest to us during the ordeal. We needed support as well as celebration on this ritualistic return to the city where our journey had begun—just as triumphant, returning defending armies need to parade through their own cities, waving flags and blowing horns in order to believe it is truly all over and they are free to walk the streets again.

We began the celebration by sending flowers to all my doctors. On the actual anniversary, we had dinner with Henri and Belinda at a restaurant where desserts look like buildings under construction—a healthful concept insofar as it guaranteed that we would never order one. Belinda arrived after Henri did, and we knew in a flash; a woman in love, confident that she is loved in return, is a magnificent and undeniable sight. They were married in August. My illness had been their bardo, the line at which they could either admit their love or continue to hide it. They chose the open air.

My sisters joined us for dinner at Juliana's and Mark's the next evening, but with misgivings. "Any time but that week, Deborah, *please*," they said. They had succeeded, finally, in going back to their own lives and, still following Dad's rules about no crying in public, wanted the bad dream to go away. So I considered it a sign of true devotion that they had agreed to this reunion even though they thought it was macabre.

We met in the parking garage under the Boston Common and walked along Charles Street together. Callie's arms were filled with lilacs, the symbol of awakening love, fresh from her garden. We got stomach cramps laughing about the new family tradition she had begun. In March, Callie had turned forty-four, but she told everyone she was forty-five, stepping right over the crack of forty-four with originality, just as she used to get out of eating peas when we were little. As we set off up Beacon Hill, our laughter fueled by mounting tension about whether this party was a good idea, I was winded in minutes. Still challenged by those hills! The group instinctively slowed down to spare me from having to ask.

As soon as we were inside the apartment, my sisters' misgivings were left in a heap with their Day-Timers. Hillery and George arrived, as usual, with bags of food that would feed Juliana and Mark for a week, when all they had requested were crackers. We gathered around the big dining-room table that had centered them all a year ago, when nothing was certain except Hillery's warm chicken soup. And Jack toasted the gathering with his usual golden, Irish tongue, observing, "We have scar tissue in each of us now. But the imperfection has created a stronger muscle."

Karen enters after I am safely under the fresh, warm sheet. A scented candle flickers and soft New Age music competes for air space with the smoky perfume. I am in a pastel cocoon, sealed off from Boston's rush and roar. I am always aware that I am one of the lucky ones who can afford massage. It rankles me that most insurance companies and many doctors don't support this noninvasive therapy. Even animals have shown cardiovascular benefits from massage. Diane Ackerman, in her luscious book *A Natural History of the Senses*, cites an Ohio experiment in which a researcher fed rabbits high-cholesterol diets and methodically petted a group of them. The result: the petted rabbits had a 50 percent lower rate of arteriosclerosis than the others. In addition to improving circulation and relieving stress, massage offers the simple gift of human touch, a strong medicine in the battle against isolation and depression, both proven contributors to second, often fatal, heart attacks within one year of the first one.

But really, how can we expect doctors and nurses to recommend massage when all they've ever known is abusing their own bodies, beginning, ironically, with the rigors of medical training? Even my superb rehab instructor at Maine Medical Center did not mention massage. She did talk about the therapeutic benefits of giving and receiving a hug now and again. But I looked around the room at people who were of the generation that did not hug, who had no one in their lives, who were divorced, widowed, isolated.

"What about massage?" I offered.

The instructor agreed heartily. Still, an introduction to massage was not yet part of the Turning Point program. And there was nervous laughter in the group when I brought it up, as though someone had just farted.

Karen begins my massage with reflexology. We are both quiet as she firmly kneads various points in my foot, believed in ancient Chinese medicine to relate to specific parts of the body. The area that corresponds to my thoracic cavity is always sore. Sometimes I have to ask her to ease up.

Ten minutes into the silence, Karen suddenly speaks, as though she is responding to something I have just said.

"Your body did not betray you, you know."

Betray me? I thought I was through with all that. But her words rivet my attention, a sign that I am not through with anything yet. The breaking of my heart-the-muscle *was* the ultimate betrayal, the body betraying itself, the self betraying the self, and how is that to be resolved?

"It saved you. Your body saved you."

I lift my head slightly and peer at Karen. She locks eyes and doesn't let me go.

"You still hold your body like you are afraid something is going to hit you."

I know she's right. I walk with my shoulders tight and raised like a window sash about to crash shut. I have seen the frozen shrug myself, in mirrors and windows. Is this what Judy means when she prods me, feeling everything from my skull to my soul? Is this why I have not yet reached a state of warm chocolate pudding?

"You do not have a weak body, Deborah. It is strong, or you would not be alive. Keep drawing on it and you will heal yourself."

Lying on my back as Karen pushes with long strokes into my thighs, I am once again on the floor of Zoe's yoga studio in Cambridge one year ago when the whole sky fell on my chest and the world changed. I see my arms outstretched, palms up, shoulders relaxed and touching the floor. My right leg is straight and the left leg is slightly bent at the knee, just beginning the setup for Reclining Marīcyāsana. Named after Marīci, one of seven seers born from the Hindu creator-god Bhrama's eye, it is a heating pose (āsana) bringing warmth to all the organs, the gentle twist like a slow fire spiraling up from a log. Zoe had said that the pose should have a relaxing effect on the shoulders by creating more freedom in the shoulder joints and relieving them of their burden. Since the shoulders bear down on the heart, she explained, if you can relieve them of burden, then the heart can ascend, finding radiance like Marīci did with the birth of his grandson Surya, the sun-god.

And then it hits me so hard that I come up gasping: Reclining Marīcyāsana evokes another age-old image, that of Christ ascending with love and forgiveness into radiant heavens, relieved of his worldly burdens, arms wide open.

For one second I am suffused with understanding; it's as though I have been hiking up a mountain and my ears have finally popped so I can hear. The pose of my physical body when death came for me had been the clue all along. Mine was the redemption story. I hadn't even realized that I needed to be saved, on that Monday like any other when a torn main artery and the protection of loved ones took all burdens from my shoulders so my heart could ascend—like Christ to the heavens, like Marīci to the sun, like Gracie in her bid for freedom.

Throughout my convalescence I have struggled with feelings of resentment over the religious urgings of my well-intentioned Christian neighbors, and so I am horrified that Christ's image has come to me with such power on a massage table. It's the sort of epiphany claimed by people who wave Bibles on street corners, people I have always shuffled past quickly, averting my eyes. Far from inspiring me to join the nearest church, however, it confirms my belief in individual responsibility—manifest in the body of Christ, the life of one good man. I agree with Gandhi who said, "We must *be* the change we wish to see in the world." Or, as Perri once said to me, leaning over the counter at the bookstore after a pious town resident made it clear that homosexuals deserved no human rights, "This is the problem I have with so many of these so-called Christians. They look to some poor dead guy on a cross, when they alone are responsible for love."

Until my heart attack, I didn't realize that I had much to learn about love. But the body is a teacher and it is to be honored like the body of Christ, amen, the embodiment of love itself with his message of individual responsibility and forgiveness, beginning with forgiveness of self.

My quiet year beside the lake had opened my eyes to the lovely and intricate patterns that lead us to moments of insight like this one, moments in which we can see that tracks in the snow are a mountain range; that the plates in the skull move to the breath of the body and that the breath is like the waves of the sea, the source of all life; that a year's seasons can contain the lessons of a lifetime; that every individual's short life embodies all of humanity's suffering, mystery, and triumph. That true healing requires touching the wounds of both body and soul. To see the patterns and end your isolation, you simply have to pay attention.

My body is strong. It did not betray me.

This year of guilty languor; of slow, minute observations of nature; of quiet contemplation; of time to be angry and move through it; of receiving and expressing love—is required by anyone seriously ill to achieve physical strength and spiritual peace. I am living proof that you cannot separate matters of the heart from the muscle, as scientific research is finally agreeing.

After my epiphany with Karen, I went downstairs from the spa to eat lunch at the New Age bookstore-café. Chewing cool, crisp lettuce has always calmed me down. But the gods weren't through with me yet.

I crossed the street to browse in a few windows before my two-hour afternoon nap. A sign in a very hip shop caught my eye: SALE. What woman can resist such provocation? And a *shoe* sale, no less. Yes, I should look for shoes that represent the new liberated me, I thought. Life is simply too short for tight shoes.

The possibilities were endless as I surveyed shoe after shoe. Who am I now? What shoes do I need? What shoes do I want? In my past life, I rarely shopped unless by catalog; I bought a few classic uniforms and they worked. I grinned, thinking: *It is the middle of the day and I am not in an office.* I swelled inside with anticipation.

"May I help you?"

The saleswoman was tall, taller than I am and skinnier, too. Her long hair was looped in dreadlocks, her skin the color of morning coffee with a little cream. Her top was skimpy, her short skirt tight with a little diaphanous overskirt. Her long legs sailed along in sexy black shoes. She went into the back room again and again, trying to find something hip that would fit my slim feet. I watched her move, leonine and fluid. She was perfectly in her moment.

But nothing fit me except a pair of shoes that strapped on. I looked at her feet and sighed. I'd probably look ridiculous dressed like her, anyway. Still, I felt apologetic for having chosen something so dull, on sale for twenty dollars.

"Having skinny feet really limits the options. All your effort and I am buying old-lady shoes I have to bolt to my feet," I said.

She folded my shoes in their box with tissue paper and did not look up as she said, so quietly that I could barely hear her, "You shouldn't make fun of old ladies. It's very lucky to be an old lady."

And she continued her packing, shaking out a bag, jiggling the box into it, absorbed in her job. She did not notice that I was gripping the counter with both hands, staring at her as if I had seen the ghost of my young mother. She did not notice that I was shaking inside from wisdom that had just escaped from the lips of a gorgeous twenty-five-year-old who had turned out to be another teacher.

She looked up and smiled, "Thank you, Mrs. Heffernan."

I smiled back as though she had not rocked my being, as though this was just another transaction in the day of a privileged woman shopping when others must work. I wanted to grab her arm and ask her how she knew this already. I wanted to pull down the neck of my jersey and show her my scar while shouting, "I know, I know! You are right! I am not sleepwalking through life with a credit card as though each second is not precious. We should all be so lucky as to be old ladies!"

I hesitated for a just a moment, then said, "Thank you for all your help."

To say more would have broken the spell. And I walked out of that store with wobbly legs and a radiant heart while she turned to the next customer.

"May I help you?"

48

JUNE 8, 1998. A year ago I was shakily, dutifully walking in circles high above Beacon Hill in the gilded cage I shared with Gracie. This week we are staying with Juliana and Mark again while I have my eyes examined to check on the ravages of amiodarone, the worst of my drugs.

Yesterday, on our way to the ophthalmologist, we ran into Marc, Torch, and Greg (the cardiac anesthesiologist who believes in kisses and prayers). I am always giddy with the doctors who saved me, shamelessly in love, a medical groupie. I cannot still the electricity that runs through me wildly and attaches me to them like a magnet. How can I ever see them as ordinary guys when I feel every heartbeat as though it's my first and last? Juliana says that this will ease with time; that taking care of people like me is their job; that I may feel unique, but what they did for me they do for many others every day. But I don't believe her for one minute. When they are near I am an exploding piñata. Candy and messy emotions everywhere. Total ecstasy.

I know. I have got to get a grip.

In the ophthalmologist's office, my eyes were pronounced nearly perfect and the doctor said I didn't have to change the weak prescription glasses that I use for movies. I asked him if he could see the vortex on my cornea from the amiodarone. He said it was a "bored" question, and it took me a wounded minute to realize that he meant "board," as in exam. He said that the amiodarone-induced deposits should not affect my sight and would disappear in time after I stop taking the drug. He didn't realize that may be never. I also received a gentle scolding for having ignored my eyes for three years. But he was young and serious and I enjoyed my call-down about good vision.

I was yellow-eyed and temporarily blind from the glaucoma exam when Jack led me from the doctor's office. He decided to play hooky for the rest of the day and we made love luxuriously in the middle of the afternoon back at the apartment. Then I shoved my bony left shoulder under his right armpit, positioned my left breast on the mattress so that the box didn't stick into my ribs, wrapped my right arm and leg around him in a fierce clamp so we would be together forever and ever, and fell into a deep sleep. I appreciated that a year ago in this very bed, no sleeping position was comfortable and lovemaking was a possibility that neither of us could imagine.

Emboldened by yesterday's good review for my eyesight, this morning I've decided to walk to a place I longed to be a year ago. I am wearing sneakers, stretchy black shorts, and a T-shirt with the tree of life silk-screened on it that my sister Leesa gave me. Before I leave the apartment, I grab the cell phone and put on the power. Just in case. I head down the hill and maneuver along Charles Street, wary of bricks that could turn my ankle and absent-minded tourists looking in windows and likely to crash into me, the walking bruise machine. In the city I still feel as though I am paddling a canoe against a rushing current—people, signs, and streetlights are in full, dangerous focus as I navigate any place other than my home. All along Charles Street I search for Marvin, who prayed me back to life while he begged for spare change. Nowhere. In fact, we've never seen him again, though I look for him every time I am on Charles Street.

I cross Storrow Drive using the pedestrian bridge. Traffic buzzes beneath me, some exiting onto Cambridge Street as I once did, hurtling in an ambulance to Mass General.

Instead of turning left toward the tunnel where Jack's headlights had illuminated a green-clad person pumping my chest behind smoked glass windows, I turn right toward Boston Harbor. The ocean spices the air. I hear a muffled voice on the water and see a Boston Duck Tours boat slowly purring along, filled with tourists. Slender cormorants dive for unsuspecting fish. Roller skaters whiz by. Sinewy, tanned mothers run with babies in exercise strollers. I pass the schizophrenic woman I used to watch from my hospital window. She is walking in a leisurely fashion, sometimes pausing to talk quietly with an invisible friend or to peer into trash barrels with the discriminating eye of a Beacon Hill matron shopping at the local market.

The tennis courts are empty on this workday, a clearing in the middle of a forest of tall buildings. I think about my work sometimes. I do not miss it any more than I missed Algebra II when I'd graduated from the eleventh grade. While I had finally achieved my A in algebra, I never really understood it. And so it was with my time in corporate America. I would never have returned to who I really am if my main artery hadn't dissected and taken out my bridge—forcing a new direction. Most people would not see this as a good trade, but I do.

I round a bend and there is my corner of the Ellison building tucked behind a brick wall of Mass Eye and Ear. I count floors and calibrate the view I once had from all angles of Ellison-8, room 36.

And then I find it. I increase my pace, swinging my arms defiantly. *Show-off!* I give a big wave.

Perhaps Torch is doing his rounds, Coke can in hand, white mask loose around his neck as he lumbers down polished halls in hissing booties after another sleepless night. Perhaps Marc is struggling to get into a white jacket two sizes too small for him, simultaneously dictating the details of someone's survival into his tape recorder. I see Doreen and Joanne in the SICU monitoring blinking machines and comforting hallucinating patients. I imagine Greg expertly administering anesthesia, and Jeremy bent over a white sheet, delicately implanting another defibrillator while listening to Pablo Casals.

I imagine Debbie and Wendy delivering pills in pleated white paper cups or giggling in the shower with a delighted patient having her hair washed. I imagine Eric going home to his five children after another night of watching over people too sick to know that he is real and not a floating green shirt. There is Stan making someone laugh at a photograph of himself running the Boston Marathon wearing his Groucho mask. Miss Aida is delivering breakfast, rocking from side to side, a living lullaby. And here comes Keith to teach another person how to walk while swinging her arms and lifting her feet. I see them all with unbounded gratitude and love that fill my half-a-heart with light.

Perhaps there is another family sleeping on the floor of the SICU waiting room, stealing showers and writing in their own notebook, recording a journey of the heart that has only just begun. Perhaps someone is sitting in my chair right now—slumped over and stabbing fruit with a fork, taking the whole morning to eat a few bites, wanting so badly to breathe fresh air that smells of the sea. My wave is most vigorous for her because I have reached the point she cannot yet imagine.

I shout, "You can do this! Look at me: I am *here*. Eat your vegetables."

The crazy lady pauses in her foraging and stares at me as though I am mad.

"Life will always be without a natural, convincing closure. Except one," wrote Richard Ford. Yet that day, that splendid day of being alive on the Charles River esplanade felt like fitting closure to the end of my first year of recovery.

I look back on that year as though I lived under a spell; and anyone I've ever spoken with who has *consciously* healed after illness, the death of a loved one or another form of major loss, says the same thing. I respect that this degree of attention to every moment of one's own existence, finding meaning everywhere like Easter eggs, may be foreign to some people because they have not had life snatched away. Or if in facing loss they cannot admit their vulnerability for one reason or another. All I know is that, stripped of the ability to rely on your body, you reconstruct your life in minute detail, beginning with observing your own breath. My eighty-four-year-old friend Mim, who is struggling with cancer, describes the process as "taking one breath at a time because you cannot take two." And this seems truer and more helpful to me than similar expressions about steps (hopping on two feet works) and days (much too long to get through).

Torch once wrote us a note saying that he felt privileged to be a part of this story. *I assure you, Torch, the privilege is mine. All mine.* I would not trade the journey I am on now for the track I was on before. Sure, I would have preferred an easier route to enlightenment—and my life will continue to be seriously restricted. But if you accept that death is part of life, as I learned from this experience, then living with it every day means living fully. My future is really no more uncertain than anybody's.

Shooting stars, snatches of conversation overheard on the street, puddles reflecting the sky—these things are no longer just for me. After all, one cannot keep up that level of attentiveness, or a quick trip to the store for bread could starve a family. I will work hard, however, at maintaining the focus that has brought my heart peace. My year of healing both body and soul has taught me that concentrating on oneself for a while is not selfishness, as the circumstances of my upbringing had led me to believe; it is our responsibility. As expressed by a prayer often said after yoga practice: "May the peace I cultivate in my heart help cultivate peace in the world." I had to go to Oz and back to finally understand this, though I have seen the movie at least twenty times.

Is there a scientifically proven relationship between the state of the emotional heart and the muscle? It truly doesn't matter to me anymore because there is one thing that I do know: I explored the question and am better for it.

And I am a student of impermanence now. Things will change, have already changed, and are changing again. Someone very wise said that the longest and greatest journey is from the head to the heart. My heart attack has taught me to be patient with the journey as impermanence continues to challenge what I learned during that long, hard year. But one year is no time at all for a little enlightenment when you consider that it takes 13 billion years for the light of the stars, the edge of our observable universe, to reach us.

Epilogue

The Second Year

In September 1998 we celebrated Jack's sixtieth birthday as I'd been planning for three years—in the Alaskan bush, reuniting Jack with his two favorite climbers, Morrie and Carl. Twenty years before, Carl and his wife, Kirsten, an audiologist and a nurse, had turned their lives upside down and headed for the bush with a penny in their pockets and dreams of a self-determined life. Starting modestly with a small log cabin, they expanded the cabin into a lodge, and eventually built a network of hunting and fishing camps. Of course, in making my proposal to Marc, I emphasized their medical training. I knew he'd say no, but thought there was no harm in asking.

Miraculously, Marc approved the adventure with specific parameters: we were to remain at all times near the camps; carry oxygen; keep to my routines; have a medical network at the ready; and we were not to fly in unpressurized planes above 7,000 feet. His rationale: I would be transported faster by bush plane, Alaska's family van, to a hospital in Anchorage than I would be by ambulance to Maine Medical Center in Portland.

"It would be good for you, for both of you," he said.

So we cashed in my frequent-flyer miles, the legacy of years of commuting to Detroit, and I got to fly in the copilot's seat of a single-engine Cessna floatplane. We gazed down at Anchorage's buildings flung about like crates of Klondike supplies, at sweeping fields of red-dening blueberry bushes, dark green bear bush sculpted by the wind into formal Italian gardens, and sprays of tiny ponds like mirrors on a Rajasthani skirt. On Jack's birthday, we were four hundred miles from the next cabin under a black sky and dazzling stars with old friends tucked into their bunks and a young family of grizzlies wandering the camp. (Needless to say, I exercised indoors by jumping up and down and marching back and forth across the cabin. And we went to bed each night with rifles, mace, and two-way radios.) Most important of all, I saw Denali, The Great White One—the mountain that had trained my husband in survival all those years ago, preparing him for the test of his life on Aconcagua and mine at Mass General.

In Vancouver afterward, I slept for three days straight—but don't tell Marc.

In December, I am at Mass General for the annual test of my defibril-lator in the electrophysiology lab, followed by a checkup with Marc. I am dreading it. Paddles will be all over me, just in case, but I will never get used to this brief death and resurrection.

They were careful to schedule the draining test of my box after my pulmonary test, so I see Tatiana first. She is chatty and I enjoy her Russian accent straight out of a spy movie. I learn a lot about a televi-sion show that she watches on crime. It makes her scared to think that these things go on in the United States, but she watches it anyway, fascinated. I understand this no better than I understand why people watch shows about hospitals or disasters, given the excitement avail-able in real life.

I blow and blow and blow, my lips stretched taut in a grotesque smile around the rubber mouthpiece. I pass with flying colors and feel that a gold star should be pasted on my forehead. Lungs hold-ing steady! Though they test below normal, the amiodarone and extra exertion haven't compromised them yet.

About to dress for my stroll to the EP lab, and already feeling extremely anxious, I am apprehended by a nurse who says that now I am to undergo a stress test to measure my ejection fraction and oxygenation capacity.

This is an ugly surprise. It means I will undergo two emotionally and physically taxing tests back to back. I feel my chin quivering. *Get a grip, Deborah.* I pad into the waiting room in my johnny and hospital socks to get Jack. He is reading his *New York Times*, glasses sliding down his nose. One look and he is back in it with me.

"How did this happen, baby?"

"I don't know. I scheduled everything they told me to. They say I have to pedal a bike and I don't have sneakers, shorts, I haven't eaten . . ." (Patients are required to fast before the box test.)

I am in a panic. When I face a test, I want to get an A. For some reason, it does not occur to us to refuse to do this today.

They find me johnny bottoms and I wear my old navy low-heeled pumps that match the long skirt I chose to hide the bruises all over my legs. A nurse inserts an IV into my right arm. I feel the familiar burn and the nausea rising. Then I climb onto a bicycle seat and press my chest up against a large torpedo while extending my arms to grasp twin handles on either side of it. Once again I breathe into a mouthpiece. They deactivate my box with a flat cloth magnet and—*oh my God, will I die if they turn off my box? Will this be the moment the arrhythmia returns?*—they put defibrillator pads on my back and chest. Just in case. The doctors are new to me. One is a pulmonary specialist, and I try to calm myself by learning all I can about what that is before they tell me to start pedaling. Jack has been invited to the show and he coaches me from behind, eyes damp at the sight of his skinny wife pinned against a cold machine, holding on for dear life and pumping like hell in her ladylike shoes.

But in my head I am winning the Tour de France, out in front of the pack. What the other racers don't know is that my life depends on this race.

Surely my ejection fraction has improved. It must have. Look at me go!

It hadn't budged.

My EF measured 24 again, and my oxygenation function was that of someone twenty years older. And I would most likely be stuck with these numbers until I began the descent into congestive heart failure, the next step in my cardiomyopathy, since there is no cure for damaged heart muscle. Yet.

We crashed again.

A few weeks later my friend Ann wrote me one of her pep notes. At sixty-nine, she took umbrage at my grief.

"You will lose friends and influence with remarks like that, young lady," she wrote, reminding me that Jack was sixty and behaved like a puppy—as does she, I might add. Suddenly my leap to a virtual sixty-six seemed just fine.

Besides, in spite of the numbers, I had my own evidence that I was making progress. I was no longer the center of my own attention. And I had shifted from being strictly mono-task (brushing my teeth had been a full-time activity) to doing several things at once. Furthermore, I was losing my frozen attentiveness, a requirement if I was to survive crossing the street in traffic. Every horn no longer made its own distinct sound to be pondered for a while, slowly. The world's sights, sounds, smells were beginning to blend into the background. Perhaps best of all, I no longer heard and felt every beat of my heart; I trusted that it would work for me without my supervision. I accepted that another day would come, that every spot of light on every geranium leaf didn't need to be recorded so as not to cease to exist. I knew, in spite of the scientific data, that I was okay; I could lead this life. After all, I had been to Alaska.

Even with the memory of Alaska and his past therapy sessions with Dr. Ned Cassem, however, Jack struggled to accept the shadows in our life. My test results that December only proved to him that his guard duty was not over, would never be over. He crashed again, silently, privately, getting that vacant look in his eyes.

It's a warm, sparkling winter-into-spring Maine day, and Jack is circling me in a slow trot as I puff my way up the small incline, swinging my arms, walking as fast as I can, breathing rhythmically. Jack is beautiful to watch as he runs ahead of me, loping gracefully, slightly bowlegged, long and loose, my marathoner.

"Are you all right?" he asks.

I smile and nod. The air is crisp, the sun is warm, and I am with my love. I am very fine.

He comes up behind me and tweaks my butt, then pulls ahead of me as he does every day. Usually he turns around after a few feet and circles back. This time he goes a little farther than usual.

My heart rate is decreasing because I am going downhill now. My monitor is strapped under my sports bra, and its companion watch is beeping at me, telling me that I've slid below my minimum rate of 94. I walk faster to get it up again. My target rate is still a pathetic 94 to 98 beats a minute. For an athlete, this is barely moving. For me, it's a major workout and I'm sweating under my fleece jacket as my heart rate creeps up to 101 beats a minute. This is still considered in range.

Looking up from my watch, I see Jack ahead of me in his wool cap and mittens nearing the intersection where we usually turn around and head back. He approaches the turn and gives a tiny glance over his shoulder as he hangs a left and is out of my sight. More important, I am out of *his* sight.

Minutes go by as I approach the corner, alone for the first time ever in our post-MI workouts. As I turn left to follow Jack, I see him running ahead of me toward the farm stand where we buy carrots in summer. Jack still doesn't look back and I can feel how hard that is for him because I am on his rope.

Stay steady, my love, and don't look back. It's your turn.

And he keeps running. I feel myself begin to smile, a slow, wide grin that never stops—reaching up to the sun, lassoing a cloud.

It begins as an ordinary Wednesday. Since I no longer operate with a calendar and whole days drift by on my pillbox with no date attached to them, I do not notice the date. Today is simply the morning of my weekly yoga class.

At seven forty-five I hop in my red truck and drive up the hill, parking with the devoted few. We mill about the foyer for a while, greeting each other, taking off our socks, gathering our sticky-mats. Then we take our places facing Scott. My place is in the middle of the back row, where no one can see me falter and I focus better knowing that.

We begin as we always do, standing with our eyes closed in

Tādāsana, or Mountain Pose, focusing on our breathing. We then do interminable standing poses, lifting our kneecaps, keeping our hips back and aligned under our torsos, reaching for a distant imaginary horizon, feeling lighter and lighter. My legs are beginning to tremble, a sign that the class is drawing to a close. Then Scott instructs us to lie on our backs with our arms out to either side, palms up, our legs stretched out in front of us.

"Now bend the left knee and draw it gently over the right leg, holding it lightly with the right hand as you keep your shoulders relaxed on the floor to open your chest . . ."

Only then do I realize that it is May 12, 1999—two years to the day from the yoga class that changed my life—and that Scott is moving us into Reclining Marīcyāsana, the gentle twisting pose I was in when my heart exploded. I have not dared the complete pose since I lay on Zoe's polished Cambridge floor. Scott has never taught this pose before, nor have I told anyone in my class about its significance in my life. Weeping silently, I am grateful for my back-row sanctuary, grateful to be *alive.*

I will leave you here, as I breathe into the heart-opening pose that began my unexpected journey of the heart. In yoga, a pose is never fixed or static. Beginning each pose by breathing gently, we trigger the Relaxation Response in our bodies, the antidote to the Stress Response of "fight or flight." As the breath releases tension that we may hold within, whether from a day or a lifetime, the body relaxes further, elongating, expanding, and resolving the pose. The mind grows more peaceful, more present—awake. Yoga is a metaphor, although to an onlooker it may appear that the practitioner is doing nothing more than sprawling on the floor. A yoga pose like life, like illness, is dynamic. It is where I practice impermanence. Every day. Because things will change. They always do.

Other adventure stories tell of mountains conquered and oceans crossed by explorers who come right back home to the truth that lies within each and every one of us. My involuntary adventure in cardiac land may lack the roar of storms and fire, but it is no less epic, if you think about it. We are all Odysseus longing for Ithaca, that mythical city that is a stand-in for our true selves. Today in a world in which one tweet can begin a righteous revolution or destroy a child's reputation, perhaps our most important exploration is a quiet one, an inward journey. Our greatest responsibility may be to resolve our own pain and confusion so that we do not inflict those on others and on this precious earth. An unexamined life can be a dangerous thing, as any good biography eventually reveals about the lives of our leaders, mere mortals, just like us.

My first year in the monastery of illness gave me time to examine, understand, accept responsibility for, forgive, and heal wounds formed from the slings and arrows of my own small life. By making the effort to heal all of me, not just my body, I marshaled the strength every human has within to survive joyously—even as I limped along with half of a functioning heart, with a heart transplant in my future. In illness I discovered a vitality that I had no idea I possessed. Today, every day, I feel like a happy pre-schooler who hears her name for the first time in a roll call and excitedly shouts, "HERE!"

Yes, I am more present than I have ever been in my life, but I am not kidding myself. My cardiovascular disease is not cured. It will never go away and leave me alone. Instead I have discovered, in the words of Dr. Dean Ornish, "Healing may occur even when curing is not possible. Curing is when the physical disease gets better. Healing is a process of becoming whole."

Now, I know full well that you may have four lively young children, two jobs, migraine headaches, aging parents, and no way to simply drop out of the rush and roar as illness forced me to do. This book is my way of joining your tea party that I mentioned in the Prologue. I am your CliffsNotes. Use my experience as encouragement to pay attention to your own life, to the beat of your own precious heart. How do you really want to live this short life? Begin now by, say, eating an apple and really enjoying it. Increments matter. Small steps are how all worthwhile change is accomplished.

As the years progressed, I have remained a keen and often baffled student of impermanence. One ICD was soon exchanged for another. Drugs and dosages were adjusted. Side-effects compounded and compromised other parts of my body. Lots of blood was drawn and tested.

More scars formed and thickened. I became spotted with purple bruises from the blood thinners. I had good days and bad days. But every morning, there I was on my yoga mat at the foot of our bed.

Most people dream of a delicious dinner with their one true love. Jack and I feasted at this banquet every single night—even as I grew thinner and paler. Jack insisted that I was beautiful. I worried about the tension around his eyes. He would not talk about it, and continued coming up with inventive ways for us to enjoy this life. We even traveled, breaking out of our corral only for places with sophisticated medical systems. Every day I ate consciously, loved completely, and collapsed into sleep for a few hours in the afternoon. Then I woke and walked with Jack as far as I could. Often I could not. If I was crabby, I did my best to apologize. And then I forgave myself, most of the time.

Jack retired, or as we call it "graduated." His hair turned white in Irish fashion, but his smile remained a beacon. Silver hairs multiplied in my unruly mane, now thinning from poor vascular circulation. I acquired distinct wrinkles around my eyes. My underarms jiggled, appalling me. I was aging along with the rest of my peer group, but vanity meant I was still alive.

My father and Jack's mother died, making us all very sad and altering family dynamics once again. Our families took their turns stumbling, struggling, and triumphing. We grew to appreciate them all even more. We laughed a lot. Marriages were celebrated or ended, more grandchildren were born, and our magical niece Clara was adopted all the way from China.

Friends went through their own changes: moving, divorcing, switching jobs or retiring, remarrying, traveling, fighting cancer, receiving knee replacements, learning to dance. Wars were waged, economies rose and fell and rose and fell. Politics infuriated. Jack and I became even more engaged locally, the only place most of us can make a difference. Meanwhile, our gardens expanded and matured with chaotic beauty, as Lucia and I became even more honest with ourselves about which plants will thrive on this windy point and which ones will not.

All these changes took place and more, and Jack and I participated—limited only by frequent commutes to Mass General and my daily routine of drugs, exercise, and increasing fatigue. Heart failure determined the schedule of our life together, but it did not determine its quality. It has never defined me. With time my illness, its rhythms and demands, became like the tick of a clock that only Jack and I could hear.

Marc continued to see a heart transplant in my future, but Jack could no longer get him to commit to a deadline, because I passed a few of those against all odds. Instead, Marc left my future as wide open as the sky—at least that is what I chose to hear.

Then the future arrived, as all futures do. Nine years after my first astonishing MI, the right coronary artery (RCA) dissected following a gentle massage. Go figure. There was no recovering from this blow. Now I slept for most of the day. Six months later on August 21, 2006 I gratefully received a heart transplant at Massachusetts General Hospital. Today I am thriving with the heart of a perfect stranger—but that is another story entirely.

By the way, those two apple saplings that Jack planted on our point among the huckleberry bushes and granite boulders? They struggled along for awhile, doing their genetic best to survive in an environment that did not support and nurture them. Ultimately they did not make it. But I did, in good part because I am exactly where I belong.

Women's Heart Attack Symptoms and Support

The most common heart attack symptom for both women and men is chest pain or discomfort. Other symptoms are more subtle—like shortness of breath, nausea/vomiting, and back or jaw pain—and are often women's only symptoms. Do not dismiss these other symptoms as perhaps a flu coming on, or a little stress or indigestion. Pay attention. For me, the most important signal was a voice that whispered within me that "Something is very, very wrong." That voice of intuition saved my life. Do not deny your intuition if you feel any of the following:

- Uncomfortable pressure, squeezing, fullness, or pain in the center of your chest that lasts more than a few minutes, or goes away and comes back

- Pain or discomfort in one or both arms, the back, neck, jaw, shoulders, or stomach

- Shortness of breath or difficulty breathing—with or without chest discomfort

- Clammy sweat, nausea, or feelings of lightheadedness, dizziness

- Unusual fatigue or weakness, especially with exertion

- Unexplained feelings of anxiety or "impending doom"—a sense that something is seriously wrong in your body.

If you think you are experiencing a heart attack

1. **Call 9-1-1, because YOU matter.** Follow the operator's instructions. You are doing the right thing by calling for help; you are not creating a fuss. It is tragic that when women experience heart attack symptoms, they are less likely to call 9-1-1 for themselves than they are for someone else, according to the American Heart Association.

2. **Take an ambulance to the nearest hospital.** Do not drive yourself or have someone else drive you, unless you have no choice. If this is a heart attack and it unfolds in transit, you will want to be with professionals who know how to save your life.

3. **Thoroughly chew and swallow a chalky aspirin—without water.** An aspirin thins your blood and may prevent dangerous clotting. Chew more than one aspirin, however, and you risk stomach bleeding.

4. **Stay calm.** It helps to take deep, slow breaths while you wait for emergency responders. Gently activate your Relaxation Response throughout your ordeal.

5. **Be direct in your communication:** "I think I am having a heart attack." This mobilizes everyone quickly. Just a bad case of indigestion from too much pizza? Everyone in the ER will celebrate your good fortune! You did the right thing by taking your life seriously.

6. **Be sure that your hospital gives you a complete cardiac evaluation, including a blood test to check your cardiac enzymes and an electrocardiogram (EKG).** As one EMT told me, "Today, if something is going on between a woman's jaw and her hip bone, the first thing we do is check for a heart attack."

My favorite websites for information and support

The following national organizations have local chapters and uncommonly helpful people:

- www.GoRedForWomen.org: the website for The American Heart Association that is focused on women and cardiovascular disease

- www.WomenHeart.org: the website for The National Women's Coalition for Women with Heart Disease.

Are You a SCAD Survivor?

Years after my first dissection and well before my second, I ran into one of my favorite boyfriends in the corridors of MGH, Michael Jaff, DO, a leading vascular specialist and Chair of the hospital's Institute for Heart, Vascular and Stroke Care.

"I keep thinking about your case, Deb," Michael said, still puzzling long after I had given up hope of ever knowing *Why me?*

"This is the best that I can come up with. It may have been a genetic defect in the collagen of your LAD. But this is just a guess."

That educated guess may be all I will ever know. At the time of my first MI, I seemed to be one of a few isolated cases of spontaneous coronary artery dissection in the US. No one was offering any better explanation even nine years later following the dissection of my RCA. Though occasionally contacted by other women who had dissected in their prime—ranging from a young mother in Ireland to a sturdy cowgirl in Montana—I did not think of *Arrow* as a dissection story, because I had concluded that we were freaks of nature. Wrong. Now we know that while surviving a dissection is rare, experiencing one happens more often than we would like to think. Furthermore, men can dissect, too!

Today we actually have a name, SCAD! a.k.a the SCADS or SCADsters. More importantly, research on our predicament has finally begun. Still, aside from the obvious connective tissue disorders, no one to date has come up with a proven common cause for our dissections. Technically I am no longer a "SCAD member," because a new heart comes with all the plumbing. But I remain keenly interested in developments. You can find links to the websites/research programs for SCAD that I know about on my website (www.deborahdawheffernan.com or www.arrowthroughtheheart. com). I will do my best to keep information updated, because impermanence rules in all matters. If you are one of the lucky ones, the few SCADs who have survived, I urge you to identify yourself to these programs. Together, we just might learn, *Why me?*

- www.scadalliance.org: This is my favorite group. The SCAD Alliance website is kept up-to-date with information about all SCAD efforts; in fact, they kindly provided most of the website addresses below. The SCAD Alliance raises awareness as well as funds for research at any qualifying institution.

- www.scadresearch.org: A terrific website begun in 2011 following the death of the founder's wife, SCAD Research largely funds the Mayo Clinic's groundbreaking program.

- The Mayo Clinic in Rochester, MN: www.mayo.edu/research/ centers-programs/spontaneous-coronary-artery-dissection-scad/overview.

- Massachusetts General Hospital in Boston, MA: www.mass-general.org/heartcenter/services/spontaneous-coronary-artery-dissection.aspx for interdisciplinary research being conducted at the MGH Institute for Heart, Vascular and Stroke Care.

- Canada: www.scad.ubc.ca for research being conducted at Vancouver General Hospital, University of British Columbia.

- United Kingdom and European Union: http://scad.lcbru.le.ac. uk/node/6 for research being conducted at NIHR Leicester Cardiovascular Biomedical Research Unit.

A Plea for Organ Donation

Over 120,000 people are currently waiting for an organ transplant in the United States. Today's shortage of donated organs means that an average of 21 people die each day because an organ does not become available in time.

Currently, over 4,000 Americans need a heart transplant. About 1,500 of them are younger than 50. Each year, only about 2,500 hearts become available for transplantation. Because I am one of the very fortunate to receive the heart of a perfect stranger, I am pleading with you to Donate Life. Be sure to make your wishes clear by taking the following two steps:

1. Go now to www.DonateLife.net and register online as a donor in your state.

2. Inform your family of your wish to be a donor. It is always easier for your loved ones when they know of your end-of-life decisions.

Acknowledgments

Let's begin at the end, with the publishing process itself. There are not words enough to express gratitude to my original editor Rachel Klayman—now an editor at Crown Publishing, an imprint of Penguin Random House—who in 2002 brought *Arrow* to publication when she was an editor at The Free Press of Simon & Schuster. I liken the process of working together to weeding next to a master gardener. She helped me to identify the important plants and clear the distractions, to honor the bones of this book. As far as I am concerned, Maxwell Perkins is alive and well in the small body and large mind and heart of Rachel Klayman, whose sensitive, skillful editing helped me to sound more like myself than when I wrote all alone.

Profound gratitude also goes to my kind and savvy agent Liv Blumer, who succeeded not only in shepherding this book through one publisher, but also into its revised and updated e-version with Open Road Media. Thanks to Michael Palgon at Open Road, *An Arrow Through the Heart* will continue to save lives, perhaps in all ways.

Going back in time to the beginning of this book's publication process, I am deeply grateful to my friend Molly Friedrich and her colleagues, who gave me tough love when I needed it and invaluable

281

guidance. Very special thanks goes to "book doctor" Jerry Gross, who died in 2014. His enthusiasm for this book in its infancy and his critical editorial comments gave me the courage to work harder. Jerry was a gifted and generous teacher, as many well know. I will always regard Jerry and his wife Arlene as the book's godparents for their kindness as well as their unwavering belief in the project.

A big thank-you goes to Martha Levin and Dominick Anfuso for championing this book when it was first launched by The Free Press (sadly, now defunct) of Simon & Schuster. They and their sales, marketing, and publicity team brought this little book about love and healing into the world against the odds, in the wake of 9/11. I am especially grateful to artist Honi Werner, who designed the quietly beautiful original cover and who in retirement generously gave me permission, with her "blessings," to use her art work again in designing *Arrow*'s current cover. Blessings on you, too, Honi.

I am indebted to early critical readers, especially Elsa van Bergen and Jan Johnson Dantrell, as well as Steven Fischer, Pamela Sardeson, Maria Friedrich, Juliana and Mark Phillips, Laura Moorehead, Eve Abreu, and Barbara and Stan Cohen. Thank you to our town's Literary Critics Society, which convened only once and only for me. Its members—Perri Black, Justin and Pam Ward, and Judith Jenness—offered crucial advice and encouragement. And thank you to Scott Manning and Larry Ashmead for their wisdom.

Many people have been instrumental in getting the word out about this book, especially Matthew Bannister and Dennise Whitley of the American Heart Association, as well as the Public Affairs team at Massachusetts General Hospital.

I have made every attempt to be accurate, but any errors of fact or interpretation in this book are entirely mine. Since cardiovascular disease statistics and therapies change at a mind-boggling rate, please talk with your doctor before making decisions about your health.

Now for the many people intimately involved in my recovery. Some of the following appear in the book; most do not because publishing wisdom forced me to remove their names for fear the reader would need Cliffs Notes, as though keeping track of the characters in *War and Peace.* But their absence does not diminish the depth of their involvement during that one critical year. Though it is not fashionable to write a long list of acknowledgments, I have no choice. It is important to understand how many people—and even more who go unmentioned here but know who they are—play an important role in a patient's healing.

Thank you is such an inadequate response to someone who has saved your life. But it is all I have. So, my heartfelt thanks to:

The heroic people who became involved from the minute Jack received the phone call that would determine our entire future—Henri Termeer and Belinda Herrera Termeer, Dr. Rich Moscicki, and Dr. Mark Goldberg, all from Genzyme Corporation; Dr. W. Gerald Austen, former chief of cardiac surgery at Massachusetts General Hospital; and Dr. David Lederman, founder of Abiomed, Inc., the makers of the latest artificial heart.

The team of dedicated, talented, sleep-deprived doctors—Marc Semigran, David Torchiana, Greg Koski, Jeremy Ruskin, Hasan Garan, Tom MacGillivray, George Tolis, John Bailey, Joseph Gavin, David Keane, Chuck Carpenter, John Mills, Jim May, and Ned Cassem at Massachusetts General Hospital; Barbara Spivak and Leonard Zir at Mount Auburn Hospital; Dixie Mills of Women to Women; Carl Sze of Maine Cardiology Associates; Karen Olson of Portland, and Judy Shedd of North Bridgton, Maine.

The assisting cardiac medical team at Massachusetts General Hospital, especially Stan Wasserman, Jerene Bitonvo, Judy Rieker, Debbie Skoniecki, Wendy Oleksiak, Doreen McPherson, Joanne Sawyer, Mary Toomey, Mary McPhee, Michelle Anderson, Tony Scheim, Eric Dunkley, Denise Graham, Lucy Ettleson, Ann Lapierre, Mary Guy, Lisa Torre, Carolyn Anderson, Felice Ricardi, Sue Beth Brown, Mary Nichols, Pamela Sullivan, Cheryl Gomes, Christine McAvoy, Suzanne Vass, Katie Swigar, Stacy Finklea, Guylene Muzak, Marie Aillen, Dru Balgobin, Grace Osazee, Dottie Bowers, John Harris, Kathy Nee, Kristin Parlman, Keith Wade, Janice Walls, and Miss Aida Allen.

The assisting cardiac medical team at Mount Auburn Hospital, especially Stephanie Boyce, Grant Kelly, Kathy Jerz, Barbara Simonson, Anand Barde, Meg Morris; and the staff at Mount

Auburn Associates who assisted Dr. Barbara Spivak, especially Linda Schwalm.

Gifted practitioners of complementary medicine, especially Zoe Stewart, my yoga teacher, as well as massage therapists Toni Forsythe, Joyce Quinn, and Karen Bowen; yoga teacher Scott Davis; acupuncturists Meg Castagna and Jamie Walker.

The staff at Turning Point, Maine Medical Center's fabulous cardiac rehabilitation program, especially Kathleen Giobbi, Jeri Lynn Schroeder, Lisa Lozier, Ann Cannon, Cynthia Rubinoff-Myers, Ellie Christie, Gail Crocker, Laurie Allard, Lori O'Donnell, and Donna Chaplin-Umbro.

Loretta Ho Sherblum, who calmly helped us to sort out health insurance issues; the people of Tufts Total Healthcare Plan, who covered me without a hassle; our beloved local pharmacist, David Diller and his wife, Jo Anne; the good people at our local Northern Cumberland Hospital; George Kimball and Hal Bartke at Kimball's Ambulance Service.

The many other employees of Genzyme Corporation, especially David Kent, Bob McInerney, Jan and Christi van Heek, Duke Collier, Judy Ozbun, Jane Burdis, and Deborah Canner, as well as Arthur Telligan; friends from our residence at the Locke School condominium building, especially Jane Mann and Hugh Wright, Edith Levine, and Beverly Melby Tringale; the thoughtful staff of the Harvard Club of Boston; Susan and John Ortiz for their extensive prayer circle extending from California to Puerto Rico; and other friends, and friends of friends, around the world whose thoughtfulness contributed to my recovery and sustained Jack—people who sent flowers, gifts, and letters, which I was too weak to acknowledge with a thank-you note.

The core group of cherished old friends who rallied around us— baby-sitters, hospital-vigil holders, writers of constant notes—Hillery and George Ballantyne, Joe and Cynthia Baratta Flatley, Linda Bennett, Jamie Bennett, Ann Carlsmith, Rob and Laura Carlsmith Bast, Carin and David Cluer, Alan and Cynthia Davis Hall, Katherine "Tink" and David Davis, David and Judy Downes Davis, Dot and Tom Dwyer, Frank and Delphine Espy Eberhart, David and Ellen Feld Gibbs, Steven Fischer, Maria Friedrich and Michael McTwiggan, Pat

Giulino, Peter Kemble, Scott and Cynthia Packert Atherton, Hope Sardeson, Pamela Sardeson and her son Daniel Willard, Alma Sertel, Morrie and Michelle Sosin Trautman, Saskia Verschoof, Carol and Bob Weekes, and high-school buddy Father Fred Enman, S.J., who said an early Sunday mass for me in the same church where I took first communion, flirted with altar boys, and mourned the passing of my parents, who died thirty-seven years apart.

Our Maine neighbors, who kept an active eye on us, brought vegetables and field flowers, and took me for walks—Sharon and Dan Abbott, Juanita and Hartley Batchelder, Perri Black, Cynthia and Bill Burmeister, Gail and Sheldon Chaiken, Laurie and Bruce Chalmers, Lil Chaplin and Peg Ward, Sandra and Steve Collins, Annie Curtis, Carol and Bruce Davis, Bob and Sally Dunning and their children Jessie and Dan, Toni and Dan Forsythe, Arlene and Joe Gallinari, Olga Gallinari, Candy and Ted Gibbons, Mim Hamilton, CC Hamilton, Brooke and Ron Hatch, Bob Jayne, Barbara and Hans Jenni, Elizabeth and Glen King, Kristi and Jon Marshall, Greg Marston, Laura Moorehead and Eve Abreu, Eleanor and Norm Nicholson, Antonietta Orlandella, Rex Rounds, Christine and Alex Stevens, Misty and Brook Sulloway, Fritz von Ulmer, and Brian Grennan.

The Terry family and crew of Perennial Point of View, especially my dear friend Lucia Terry, who in saving my gardens willed me back to earth; Paul Mark Gallinari for plowing our driveway second (after that of his grandmother Olga); our ingenious alarm guy, Bill Melby; the Cook "boys," Adam and Aaron, who cleared our driveway of fallen trees during the 1998 ice storm; and many other kind citizens of our small town, from the mail carriers to the employees of the town's old A&G grocery store.

Jack's lively, kind, ninety-one-year-old mother, Marie "Mimi" Heffernan, who is the dearest friend anyone could have; the extended Heffernan family, including Jeanne and Peter Murphy, Aurelie and Gary Druckenmiller, Joan and Agnes Adams, Drs. Sue and Jardy Durburg, Lois and Bill Weber, and Rosemary Weber.

My numerous Shea and Daw cousins, especially Anne Shea Bliven for sending me French movies.

My extraordinary father, Robert Kindellen Daw (now residing in the heavens and who would not have read this book anyway because he never looked back), who bought me my first typewriter and who taught me to live with gusto and walk fast; my mother, Ann Shea Daw, who before she died at forty-four gave me her love of reading, her poems, and the simple, steadying gift of time together.

Our families, who gave us the best medicine of all—unconditional love—especially my sisters, who generously put their own lives on hold for over a year: Ann Daw, Leesa Daw, Rebecca Daw, Callie Daw Crosby and her son Christopher Crosby; my brother Rob and his wife Gina; Jack's children: Brenda Heffernan, Tim and Maura Heffernan Cronin, Walter and Mary Kate Heffernan McTeigue, Peter and Meghan Heffernan Quigley, John Heffernan, and their mother Brenda Heffernan, as well as all the grandchildren: Fiona, Wally, Simon, Sean, Cotter, Calvin, Mary, Charlie, Lucy, Declan, and Mia.

And finally Jack, my source of joy, who has saved my life in all ways.

I thank all of you from the bottom of my half-a-heart. Please eat your vegetables and walk vigorously for thirty minutes every day, reducing your chances of getting heart disease by 40 percent.

About the Author

Deborah Daw Heffernan is a graduate of Georgetown and Harvard Universities. She has worked as a teacher in Switzerland, an associate dean at Boston University, a Fellow at the National Endowment for the Arts, and a free-lance writer. For fourteen years she was vice president of a leading Boston-based corporate training/consulting firm—until a near-fatal heart attack changed her life forever. She lives with her husband, Jack, on a small lake in Maine.

Jack and Deborah Daw Heffernan donate all Deborah's book-related earnings to cardiac causes. By buying a book, you are saving a life! The American Heart Association and Massachusetts General Hospital are primary recipients. Others include The Heart Rhythm Foundation (founding contributors), WomenHeart, and The SCAD Alliance.

CPSIA information can be obtained
at www.ICGtesting.com
Printed in the USA
FFOW04n1610110117
31129FF

9 781504 009218